DO NOT REMOVE
CARDS FROM POCKET

6/5/72

UNPREPARED!

A Husband's Story of Coping
With His Wife's Stroke

Ellwyn K. Collins

with Mary Hughes, M.A.,
Constance S. Shaffer, O.T.R.

Deaconess Press
Minneapolis, Minnesota

First published March 1992

ISBN 0-925190-50-0
Library of Congress Catalog Card Number 91-077594

Printed in the United States of America
96 95 94 93 92   8 7 6 5 4 3 2 1

Cover design by Michael Smith

Editor's Note: Deaconess Press publishes books and pamphlets related to the subjects of physical health, mental health, and chemical dependency. UNPREPARED! and other publications do not necessarily reflect the philosophy of Fairview or Fairview Deaconess, or their treatment programs.

Dedication and Acknowledgments

This book is dedicated to the beautiful people who have been given little credit for their accomplishments in the world of health care: the therapists. Their dedication and abilities rival those of the doctors and nurses, and are invaluable in bringing disabled persons back to useful and enjoyable lives.

I dedicate this book to physical, occupational, and speech therapists the world over, and particularly to the following persons who are restoring a useful life to Constance, my wife. To Maare, Rachel, Rhonda, Laurie, Artie, Candice, Connie, and a host of others whose names I have forgotten, but whose efforts are certainly remembered.

Among the other health care professionals who helped Constance, I would like to acknowledge the following:

Dr. Zarling, who guided her through the first critical days of the horrible trial.

A special note of appreciation goes to Mary of Social Services and Bonnie, a Licensed Practical Nurse.

Finally, to the warm and understanding staff of Fairview Southdale Hospital in Edina, Minnesota, including the guiding geniuses who manage to make palatable meals for the patients; they deserve all kinds of kudos.

Contents

Foreword

For every action there is a reaction. Sometimes, however, the reaction is a very long time coming.

As a child, my mother would insist that I not only learn to do the dishes, make beds, and fix meals, but that I also learn to iron clothes. "You never know when you'll need to know how to do these things," she insisted.

It was not until my wife had a stroke and I was put in the role of housekeeper that I fully appreciated my mother's efforts to teach me domestic chores.

While the female caregiver of a stroke victim ceratinly has a great weight to bear, I feel that the male caregiver needs even more insight and guidance, since he will probably enter the kingdom of the kitchen unprepared and unarmed, to say nothing about the rest of the house.

Health professionals call a stroke a "cerebral

accident," perhaps for lack of a better definition. The victim, apparently healthy and robust one day, is a relatively helpless individual the next. This disease, I am told, lashes out at 500,000 people a year in the United States alone, so my story is far from unique.

When two people stand at the altar and promise to love, honor and obey in sickness and in health, the future is rosy and full of promise. When a severe health problem arises, the oath of faithfulness takes on its full meaning. This, then, is what this book is all about.

One
The "Accident"

Saturday morning began like any one of a million others, nothing different about it. Constance, Connie to her friends, but privately known to me as Const, busied herself with whatever women find necessary to fuss about when they aren't fussing over grandchildren. About noon she decided to iron a couple of pieces of wrinkle-free clothing. Moving about on the carpeted kitchen floor, she noted that she tripped slightly a couple of times. In retrospect, this was the initial onset of a very dramatic event which would change our lives.

Later that evening Const became annoyed because the count on her knitting pattern refused to come out right. I gave it no thought, since every now and then she would find a pattern that would refuse to cooperate. She is a professional at knitting and crocheting and has picked up errors in patterns more frequently

1

than the publishers are willing to admit. She finally set the project aside and contented herself with watching some TV until bedtime.

Sunday morning proved uneventful. I wandered out to the garden and then became engrossed in conversation with a neighbor. Const came out and walked about in the yard, but I could see that something was bothering her. She was restless and mentioned that she could not shake off a strange, unsettling feeling. I had no reason to believe that it was anything to be concerned about.

In the afternoon I had an appointment as a consultant to examine a project about ten miles from home. Const was willing to accompany me, and we drove out to the site. She joined in the conversation between myself and the shop owner and was busily examining the new machines when she suddenly asked if there was a place to sit down for a minute. The casualness of the request gave me no cause to be alarmed. After taking a break, she returned and joined in the discussion over the merits of the new machinery. Her questions and comments were thoughtful and incisive; Const and I ran a screen printing shop for several years, and she is an authority on the subject.

In a few minutes she excused herself again and went back to the office. When she came back she told me that she did not feel well and would like to go home. Something in her tone of voice worried me a little, but for all I knew, something she had eaten might have caused the discomfort—she told me nothing except that she didn't feel well.

We tooled down the freeway in silence, and I kept

myself busy with the heavy Sunday traffic. About halfway home, Const squirmed restlessly and raised her left arm over her head. The arm came flailing down uselessly onto the armrest. I caught the incident from the corner of my eye, but being occupied with driving, I had no opportunity to study her. A sort of warning light came on in my mind, but I had no idea of the significance of what had happened. If any meaningful conversation took place between us, I don't recall it; I was watching for an opportunity to maneuver into the right lane in order to take our exit off the interstate.

Within a few minutes we arrived home, and as I pulled into the driveway I decided to leave the station wagon out rather than put it away in the garage. Somewhere in the thickness of my skull I had the premonition that I might have an urgent need for the car before the day was over. Had I known all the facts, I would have kept right on going to the hospital.

When her arm had fallen, Const had reached up and pushed her face away from me so I couldn't see her fear. It was at this point that she discovered the left side of her face was numb, but I did not learn this until much later. At this point I only knew something was wrong, and had no idea what it was.

Once we were in the house and Const was in her favorite chair, she seemed to relax and we started to talk. Most of the conversation centered around her denial that anything major was bothering her.

I suggested that we should call the doctor, knowing full well that Sunday afternoons are a trying time to seek medical help. Being in a hospital emergency room on Sunday can be an exercise in patience. Hospitals dread the weekend rush, and sorting out the real from the imaginary problems becomes a priority in the emergency room.

"Do you want me to call a doctor?" I repeated. By now I had a feeling that something was definitely wrong.

"No," she replied, "what if I get the one I don't like?"

The clinic we use has four doctors, and after twenty years of periodically requiring their services, we had comfortably settled on one particular doctor. That is, until recently. Because of her hearing loss, Const had decided to change from our older doctor to one of the younger doctors who speaks louder. The doctor she was referring to, however, was neither of these.

"Well," I advised her, "let's call the answering service and see if they'll tell us who's on duty."

Const got on the phone, and her face lighted up as she spoke into the receiver. I knew before she told me that the doctor on duty was her newly acclaimed one and not the one she disliked. What she didn't know was that by now my concern was sufficient that it didn't matter who the doctor might be—I was determined to make the trip with her as soon as possible.

My anxiety had grown because I could see Const was becoming increasingly distraught, even though she was trying desperately not to show it for fear of upsetting me. We were now communicating by mental telepathy, it seemed.

By her responses over the phone I could tell the

4

doctor was questioning her at length about her problem. She responded by saying that it could be a touch of flu or gas. After a moment, in a very strained voice, she said what she had been denying...she was possibly in the midst of a stroke. She hung up the phone and said, "We're to meet him at the emergency room right away."

Mary Hughes is a Medical Social Worker who became acquainted with Mr. and Mrs. Collins after Mrs. Collins was first admitted to the hospital. In the following piece, and in others interspersed throughout this book, she offers professional insight into the psycho-social aspects of stroke, examining many of the issues faced by both the caregiver and the patient.

"Stroke" is a very appropriate word to describe a cerebral vascular accident (CVA). It's like a bolt of lightning that strikes a person, and it can have as dramatic an impact on the rest of the patient's life. On the day before the stroke, the person may be healthy and active. When the CVA strikes, it can leave that person with weakness, paralysis, speech and language deficits, and behavior and memory deficits.

The idea that stroke is a medical problem that only affects the elderly is a myth. Although it is more common in older people, there is no prescribed age at which a stroke can occur. There are cases of young children, adolescents, and people at every stage of adulthood who have suffered a CVA.

A stroke has a great impact on both the stroke survivor and the significant people in the patient's life. The amount of success a person achieves in taking the steps toward recovery depends to a great extent on the support he or she receives from family and friends, and how closely they work with the attending team of health care professionals in conquering the challenges that the stroke has posed.

While going through the recovery process, it is important to work on the strengths or abilities that the individual has rather than emphasize limitations or disabilities. By focusing on positive traits, the individual will learn how to become very resourceful in order to gain the maximum potential for living a happy and productive life.

There were no available places to park anywhere near the emergency room entrance. Our daughter works as an assistant in another hospital's emergency room, and had repeatedly informed us about the rash of weekend visitors with both real and imaginary problems. We might have received preferential treatment at her place, but while our doctors were allowed to practice there, they were reluctant to because the freeway all too often turned into a parking lot, and they would be of little use to anyone while caught in traffic.

I debated between leaving the station wagon in the middle of the street and driving over to a parking ramp about a block away. I selected the latter as the lesser of two evils; Const would not have approved of my parking in the middle of the drive on her behalf, and I thought it best not to agitate her.

Soon after we left the car I noticed that her left foot was starting to drag. We got to the entrance of the hospital and were greeted by a receptionist whose job it was to get all the data that the hospital required. Considering the urgency of the problem, it seemed to me that we were simply adding even more useless information to a computer file that more than likely no one would ever look at. As you might imagine, I was starting to become annoyed and anxious by this seemingly endless delay.

Eventually we were escorted into a ward, Const's condition having given her precedence over about ten other patients. As we passed an office cubicle the emergency doctor on duty looked up with a shocked expression—it was the older doctor who used to treat us. I'm certain that Const took heart in the fact that not one, but two of her doctors were right there—the younger doctor had arrived as we were providing the receptionist with the necessary information. After a brief examination by the younger doctor, who refused to speculate on a diagnosis, he went to a nearby phone and ordered a "CAT scan," or a Computerized Axial Tomography. This machine would tell the doctor what was going on in Const's brain. It wasn't until later that I would figure out exactly why this procedure was done before any treatment was administered.

There are two types of strokes. One is the type where the blood vessel suffers a blockage and denies blood to an area of the brain. The other is one where the vessel ruptures and bleeds inside the brain.

Immediate treatment for one type could destroy any chances of recovery from the other type. To treat the blockage, the blood is thinned down by medication to reduce the obstruction and possibly remove it. With the bleeding type, surgery is considered. The CAT scan would tell which type of stroke was in progress.

When a person enters the hospital with symptoms of a stroke, the first step usually takes place in the emergency room. It is here that she will first be examined by a physician, who will check neurological symptoms such as weakness, dizziness, paralysis, and problems with speech, vision, or memory. In addition, tests may be ordered, such as blood work or a Computerized Axial Tomography Scan, which I'll explain later. The emergency room physician contacts the patient's primary physician in order to report the findings and to allow that doctor to make plans to have the person admitted to the hospital.

At this stage of treatment, two things are being done simultaneously. First of all, a diagnosis is being made of the location of the stroke in the brain and the severity of the stroke. At the same time, the patient is being medically stabilized. In order to assist with the diagnostic procedures, the primary physician may call a neurologist in on the case.

In addition to the CAT, or Computerized Axial Tomography Scan, another diagnostic procedure that may be done is an MRI, or Magnetic Resonance Imaging. The main difference between these tests is their sensitivity in how an image is viewed. The MRI is more sensitive, and can view smaller areas in more

The "Accident"

detail. During an MRI, the patient lies on a table which slides into a hollow cylinder. When the machine is in operation, it makes a loud noise, like someone is drilling or knocking nearby.

Other tests that may be administered include cerebral blood flow studies and ultra sound. The nurse also does regular neurological exams.

In the first such exam, the nurse uses a small flashlight to check the patient's eyes and asks the person to squeeze a hand or wiggle toes. This is a way for the nurse to spot any changes in the patient's neurological functioning. The cerebral blood flow studies measure the flow of blood to the brain, and help to detect abnormalities. An ultra-sound may be done to observe if there has been narrowing of the carotid arteries in the neck.

To medically stabilize the patient after a stroke, there is an initial period where bedrest is required. During this time, the person is given an anticoagulant, or blood thinner, usually in the form of the drugs heparin or coumadin. Regular protime tests may be taken. This test checks the coagulation of the person's blood to determine what dose of anticoagulant medication should be given.

The immediate focus of treatment is to keep the blood circulating to the brain tissue. If the stroke was caused by a blood clot, medication is used to prevent the clot from becoming larger or recurring.

Support from family and friends is especially important during this initial phase of the stroke. It is helpful for them to obtain educational information at this time from the nurse, physician, or hospital social

9

*worker so that they can come to a better understanding
of what has happened to their loved one and be better
able to offer encouragement. Simply being present for
the stroke survivor is highly important, and visitors
should work to maintain a positive and reassuring
atmosphere. At the same time, it is important to
remember that the patient needs more rest during this
phase.*

I could see both the doctors conversing through an
office window. They were looking in our direction.
The younger one put on his most professional face
and rejoined us. I had the distinct feeling they were
both reluctant to give their preliminary diagnosis to
one of their favorite patients.

"You have a weakening on the left side," the
younger doctor said, "and we want to keep you
overnight."

The CAT scan resembled an x-ray machine, and it
determined that Const was having a blockage type of
stroke. Immediate treatment would consist of medication to thin the blood. Although we felt anything but
fortunate at the time, an MRI, or Magnetic Resonance
Image, would be taken the following day and show
the area of damage to be deep inside the brain. If the
vessel had ruptured, surgery would have been impossible.

As we left the room where the CAT scan had been
done, our daughter Barb and her husband Bruce
greeted us. Const had called Barb before we left home
to tell her we were going to the hospital's emergency
ward.

The "Accident"

Const refused a wheelchair and insisted upon walking up to the hospital room assigned to her. As we hiked along the corridors I could see her left foot was still dragging. She was not aware of this at the time, and I certainly wasn't going to bring it to her attention; I could only guess what might be going through her mind at a time like this.

She lay in her hospital bed, helpless and confused by what was taking control of her body with such alarming ferocity and speed. I suffered with her, though not really knowing how much she was hurting from all this. Fortunately, physical pain was non-existent, except for what she described as a very strange feeling in her head for a short time. It was terrifying to see her body being injured by an unseen force and not being able to do anything about it. By now she knew what was happening; she was having a stroke. A "cerebral accident," the doctor had called it.

We stayed with Const until after she had been sedated and told she would need complete bedrest. It was about ten o'clock p.m. when I kissed her goodnight.

I spent a restless night, pitching and tossing in bed. Twice I thought I heard Const calling out to me, and I reached over to her side of the bed only to find it empty. Probably only a half dozen times in our forty-three years of marriage had I slept without her at my side.

Two

The Hospital

In the many years I had known her, Const had never expressed any particular dread of a stroke to me. Not until she was in the throes of one did she tell me that she had long been afraid of such a thing happening. I have known people who admit to these kinds of fears only to fall victim to something entirely different. Her fears, unfortunately, were well founded. Both her father and one of her brothers had succumbed to the ravages of this dread disease.

While those in the medical profession can become very vague when they do not have an answer to a problem (maybe that's why they call it "practicing" medicine), they are reasonably certain as to the causes of stroke. Smoking is a culprit in some cases, to what degree is unknown.

Foods that are full of saturated fats are known to contribute to strokes. Fatty deposits build up on the inside walls of the arteries and eventually break loose to either produce a heart attack or travel up to the brain and cause a stroke.

Heredity and high blood pressure are also culprits. In my wife's case, hardening of the arteries appeared to be the major cause. To some extent, this is a normal part of the aging process. Const had smoked since she was a young woman, although she had given up cigarettes about two months before. Her blood pressure was well within limits.

I thought that perhaps if she had given up smoking a year sooner, the stroke would not have occurred, although since then I've realized that such a statement is like playing God. Her reason for giving up smoking was indicative of her character. I had been hounding her for months to quit, with no success.

One night as she climbed into bed she said, "Feel this." She placed my hand just above her navel, on a hard spot about two inches square. She had been complaining about a pain in her left side for several days.

I suggested she call the doctor for an appointment, but she ignored my advice. This was unusual, since for the most part she always seemed willing to check in with her doctor, but she must have had other things on her mind.

Several days later, she mentioned the pain to our daughter, and later on Barb called back and informed her she had made an appointment for Const to see the doctor. Const told me she was going to call and cancel it. From years of living with her, I knew that the statement was simply meant to test my opinion. I told her to keep the appointment, and this time she accepted my advice.

The doctor examined her for the pain in her side and could find no cause. Then she remembered the hard spot on her stomach and questioned him about it.

Before we knew it, he had picked up the phone and called the hospital to arrange an ultra-sound test of the area.

The next morning we went for the ultra-sound appointment. The attendant assured her it wouldn't hurt, then smeared her stomach with some jelly to help conduct the sound waves. The waves would create a picture on a monitor screen which would tell the doctor more about her condition.

The ultra-sound device is a relatively new one, used frequently to check up on babies before they are born. How anyone could read the results of this process is a mystery to me. When the picture came on the screen it looked like a mass of roiling storm clouds or perhaps a field of jellyfish floating with the tide. As we left, I truthfully assured Const I could detect nothing in the pictures to be concerned about.

The doctor called with the results the next day. He advised her to see a surgeon, and recommended one over the phone who could help her make a final decision on how to treat the problem. This surgeon had his offices in a hospital annex which was part of the same organization for which our daughter Barb worked.

Const's first move was to call our daughter and get a report on this doctor. She came back with nothing but glowing recommendations; the hospital was his life, and he practically lived there. We met with him the next day and were quite impressed. Dr. Peterson was a relaxed, quietly confident man and leisurely took the time to answer all our questions.

The lump was a weakening of an artery wall that bulged out. The artery was a major one that travels from the heart, down the middle of the stomach, and then branches out to each leg. Anything could have caused it—smoking, heredity, or perhaps a hernia. If it had to happen, though, it was fortunate that it had appeared on the outside wall, where it could be easily detected.

The surgeon spent an hour going over the causes, possible treatments and probable results. Const had the option of delaying treatment and having the ultrasound again in three months. It was unlikely the condition would improve on its own, but Dr. Peterson did not push us for a decision, and I did not voice an opinion. The operation was a major one, and Const's health was otherwise fairly good at that time. Besides, the decision was hers to make. All her questions were answered in a straightforward manner, and while he repeatedly said it was her decision, I got the distinct impression that he favored not putting off the surgery.

After we left the doctor's office, Const tested me to see if my outlook was the same as hers. While I would never have put it the way she did, she felt like she had a bomb waiting to go off in her stomach. She decided to have the surgery.

The operation was scheduled for a few days later. The morning of her surgery, Dr. Peterson arrived and in the course of conversation, asked if she smoked.

"Not anymore," she replied.

"When did you quit?" he wanted to know.

"Last night at ten o'clock." Her sense of humor was still intact. She was true to her word, though; since she would not be able to smoke for the next week anyway by doctor's orders, she took the opportunity to kick the habit for good.

During the operation a six-inch length of dacron tubing was sewn into the artery. Afterwards she was taken to intensive care.

I had cautioned the doctor that she was highly susceptible to drugs, and that half of a normal dosage would be more than sufficient for her. She was wildly out of her head for five days after the operation, until I demanded they reduce the medications for her pain. I was becoming alarmed at her hallucinations.

Once this was done, her recovery was swift and complete. She was released from the hospital a day later. I never dreamed that we'd be back in less than two months, with a problem that made the aneurysm seem almost minor by comparison.

The first day of Const's stroke had been not only emotionally exhausting, but physically tiring as well. Six hours of pacing rock hard floors can take a toll. I suppose it makes sense for hospitals to use marble, due to the amount of wear and tear their floors get, but I haven't found a pair of shoes that will overcome the nagging back pain they produce. I'll never know how the nurses stand it.

Const's last comment before I left was that she was feeling strange. I had attributed it to the medication

17

in the I.V. Little did I realize what was in store for us the next morning.

I was up and at the hospital before eight, knowing my girl was going to need all the support and comfort I could muster. When I walked into her room, I saw her lying in bed with her left arm out from under the covers in a classic stroke position, folded up high on her breast, the hand tightly closed with the thumb locked under the fingers. She appeared to be asleep, probably sedated.

I was stunned. During the night she had lost the use of her left arm and left leg, and her mouth was drooping slightly on the left corner. As I turned to head for the nurses' station, our daughter Barb and her husband Bruce walked into the room. Barb had called the hospital to ask for a report on her mother, and had been informed of the radical changes in her condition. When I had not answered our home phone, Barb had quickly located Bruce, found a baby-sitter, and set out to head me off before I discovered the awful truth by myself. She was no more than a minute too late.

Barb relied on her medical training to take over. We went back in to Const's room, and she began bustling around, trying to make her mother comfortable and saying soothing things to her. She would glance at me periodically, I suppose to see if I was in command of myself. I could only stand there silently and hold Const's hand to assure her I was at her side. It was the only comfort I could give—I was struggling with my own emotions, and I could not allow anyone else to see them.

I certainly appreciated my daughter and son-in-law's presence, and I'm sure Const did too. Over the years, Const and Barbara have formed a bond that is a delight to behold. As husband and father, I would not have been able to penetrate it even if I had wanted to. I suspect Bruce feels this unseen force as well. In this day and age, when many daughters seem to have strained relationships with their parents, I take great pride and satisfaction in knowing this bond exists between Const and Barb.

Bruce is a son-in-law to be cherished. In times of distress or need, he appears as if by magic. He has developed the art of defining his priorities and following through on any given problem until he finds a solution. I've always appreciated this quality in him.

When the doctor arrived for his daily visit, he told us that a stroke usually took about three days to progress, and that absolute bedrest was all that could be done for her at present, other than to continue the blood thinning medication they had her on. He could give us no assurances on how much permanent damage was done.

A slight droop to Const's left eye was noticeable, and she complained about a tingling sensation on the left side of her face. But her speech was only slightly affected, which was a blessing.

When speech is disturbed, the patient often becomes emotionally distraught, sometimes to the extent of crying. Then again, some stroke victims will laugh wildly with little or no provocation. We would witness a lot of this in the next few months in other stroke patients; it's called "emotional lability." While Const was more emotional than she was previously,

I do not feel this was due to the stroke, but rather a normal reaction to the overwhelming nature of what she'd gone through. "Lability" is defined in the dictionary as "liable to change; unstable." I guess that pretty much covers the state many stroke victims find themselves in.

When it came time for the MRI, I stood outside the room where it was taking place. The machine filled the room and had a tunnel in the middle of it. Const had been placed on a table that could slide in and out of the tunnel. The operator had briefed both of us on what would take place, cautioning that when in operation, the machine would emit banging noises like someone hammering on a half-empty oil drum, only louder. They sounded more like explosions to me.

My heart went out to my wife. She suffers from claustrophobia, and that tunnel was the ultimate torture chamber for someone who dreads being closed in. She had been given a mild sedative for just this reason. The testing took less than an hour, and a medical assistant invited me into a small waiting room with a TV in it, asking if I would like to view a videotape on strokes and the care of victims.

I'm an engineer by profession, and I learned long ago that to succeed in this job, you need to have an inquisitive disposition. Fortunately, I've never been lacking in this respect, so I was naturally curious about what the video could tell me. Moreover, I had the feeling I should learn as much as possible to protect and help Const through whatever the future might bring.

Before I describe what I learned from the video, I should let you know that I have not collaborated with a medical person in the writing of my portion of this book. Medical journals are available for readers who want nothing more than a clinical approach. My intent is to provide you with an idea of some of the problems and results when the queen falls ill for a protracted time and the drone takes over in the home, and the medical information I provide is simply a layman's understanding.

The TV program was only five minutes long, but it gave me some insight into what was happening. This is what I found out:

The brain separates the control of the extremities into two halves. Damage on the right side of the brain affects the left side of the body, as in my wife's case. Left side damage—right side of the body.

Depending on which side of the brain is damaged, certain afflictions manifest themselves. Right side damage often leaves the patient visually impaired, cutting off half the vision, while this rarely occurs with left side damage. Speech can be affected by an injury on either side. Const had right side damage, so the left side of her body was affected.

Nurses and doctors can be very non-committal. Not knowing much about the affects of strokes on either side of the brain, I did not know if she had been better or worse off for having it happen on the right side. My concern for her was growing more acute with every passing hour.

Although it is more common in older people, a stroke can happen at any age and at any time. In

Const's case it came on slowly, over a three day period. More often than not, however, it happens very suddenly and without any warning.

Barb and Bruce rejoined me outside of the MRI room, intent on lending additional moral support. We found, however, there was little to be said during the next couple of hours while we waited for the results of the test.

B.J. (my name for Barb) had brought some books with her for me to read, and she wanted me to familiarize myself with their contents. Glancing at the covers, I could see they dealt with caregiving. I promised I would read them, but not right away. Just looking at the titles was enough to forewarn me that a long road lay ahead.

But if I had a long road ahead of me, what about Const?

Three

The Big Move

By Wednesday morning both Const's mouth and eye were back to normal. This improved her mood somewhat, and she probably hoped against hope her arm and leg would respond soon. At about the middle of that morning, the first knight in shining armor entered our fortress of despair. A beautiful young lady with gleaming white teeth and a slight southern twang introduced herself as "Connie" and said she was our therapist. I was not aware we had been assigned one. As she perched on the bed and began exercising Const's left arm, she informed us that a different woman would be there in the afternoon to work on her foot and leg.

This was our first knowledge that something could be done for a stroke victim. One of my old golf buddies had had a stroke and was helplessly confined to a wheelchair, and I had just assumed no help was possible for the condition. Connie manipulated Const's arm and hand gently while she talked not only to us but to the affected area. She finished after about a half hour and said she would be back in the morning. She stressed the need for caution in handling someone in my wife's condition.

Const was not to overdo things or wear herself down by performing these exercises unsupervised. Also, since the paralyzed arm weighed about fourteen pounds, she must never allow anyone else to manipulate it for any reason other than for therapy. Any physical stress on the left arm would be enough to pull it loose from the socket. The muscle tone was completely gone, and every muscle required specific attention. Do you have any idea how many muscles it takes just to scratch your nose?

It struck me as odd when the therapist started talking to Const's hand and arm, until she explained that with the slow deliberate movement, the brain not only responded to the movement, but followed the directions she was giving it! Perhaps the most amazing demonstration was when she gently tapped the muscle in Const's forearm about three times, and the wrist responded. Tapping gently in another spot, the arm responded. In this moment of enlightenment, I saw a look on Const's face that I knew well. Her eyes were flashing as she announced, "I'm going to beat this thing!"

Of this I had no doubt. The ball now rolled into my court; it was up to me to respond with equal determination. "Honey," I managed, "depend on me to give you all the help and support I can."

Later in the afternoon another therapist came in, and with hardly an introduction sat down on the bed and went to work using the same procedures on Const's foot and leg. Tap, tap, tap, and some movement, all the while talking in soft tones to the leg/brain.

The fact that Const was encouraged by these first therapy sessions was reflected by her responses when she was asked to help fill out a questionaire. When asked how much recovery she expected, she replied "All of it." While I'm sure the doctors approved of her response, I imagine they doubted her ability to attain this goal. I might have as well, if I didn't know Const.

Once the person is medically stabilized and the acute phase of the stroke is completed, it is imperative that the stroke survivor get involved in a therapy program as soon as possible. The sooner the rehabilitation begins, the better the chances for regaining as much function as possible.

The rehabilitation team includes the physicians, nurses, therapists, social worker, family members, and most importantly, the stroke survivor. The physician indicates the types and amount of therapy needed according to what the patient is able to tolerate, and monitors progress.

Depending on the person's physical needs after a stroke, the patient may be involved in one or all of the three areas of therapy: physical, occupational, and speech. The physical therapist works on the gross motor skills of the person, including ambulation, such as getting in and out of bed and moving from a sitting to a standing position. The physical therapist will also introduce a range of motion exercises for the upper and lower body extremities. If a cane or walker is needed, the recommendation comes from the physical therapist.

The occupational therapist works with the fine motor skills and the cognitive/perception skills of the individual. Some of the tasks in occupational therapy may include working on safety in activities of daily living (such as cooking), dressing and feeding skills, responding to an emergency, simple mathematical tasks, and visual and perception skills. The speech therapist works with individuals who have speech and language deficits, cognitive perceptual deficits, and problems with swallowing.

It is one of the responsibilities of the nurse as part of the rehabilitation team to assist the patient when needed and encourage as much independence with self cares as possible. The nurse serves as an educator and supporter to the patient and family. In addition, the nurse assists with the physical cares, including bathing, grooming, bathroom tasks, medical treatment, administration of medications, and the overall case management of the patient's care. The nursing personnel work with the patient twenty-four hours a day during hospitalization.

The task of the social worker who is assigned to the rehabilitation team is to serve as a support and resource person to the patient and family. The social worker will connect the patient to community resources that best meet the stroke victim's needs while working through red tape with the medical insurance provider.

Naturally, the stroke survivor takes on the most active role in the rehabilitation team. It is the patient's task to work with all the professionals and carry out the steps necessary to the recovery process.

I went home that evening and rummaged through the refrigerator for whatever might have gotten past my notice yesterday. As I sat back into my easy chair, Sam, our big black cat, stretched lazily in Const's chair and looked over my cold beans and sliver of summer sausage before deciding he could do much better outside. As I got up to let him out, the phone rang.

I am not a devoutly religious man, but a prayer slipped from my lips as I picked up the phone, fearing more bad news. It was my beautiful bride of forty-three years, and she was excited. She had managed to wiggle her index finger a little bit!

This was encouraging, but the more I thought about it, the more I looked forward to seeing it myself. It was just possible that she had wanted to start on the road to recovery so badly that she was imagining it. However, I put as much excitement as I could into my voice as I spoke to her.

The next morning I hurried to the hospital and had hardly walked in the door before she was showing me her accomplishment. I had to watch closely to see anything, but it did move.

The little finger has the smallest muscles in the human body, and the smaller the muscle, the longer it usually takes to recover. Perhaps this was a sign from above, but such a small one! By the following day the movement improved a bit, to the point where it was obvious. We were on our way.

Two days later a volunteer strode into the room pushing a wheelchair. "Mrs. Collins?" He looked at the woman in the next bed.

"Here," Const replied. "What do you want with me?"

"My name is Joe, and I have orders to bring a beautiful young lady down to therapy." His broad grin belied his age. He was enjoying retirement the best way he knew how: helping others.

I later learned that Joe had been doing volunteer work in the hospital for the past two years. The position was not unlike that of a Candy Striper. These volunteers had on plain blue coats to identify them. Almost all were retired and had a need to utilize their time in a meaningful way. Pleasant and articulate, they knew their way around the hospital and did escort service and other chores to free up the hospital people for more technical things. The volunteers did not get paid and they most certainly had to be spending their own money for transportation.

Joe wheeled us to the private elevator and brought us to the basement. We rolled into an area where Const was pushed up to a table and yet another therapist, smiling and confident, began a half hour of arm exercises, helping Const do things like push a rag in a fan-like motion over the highly polished surface. I could see it was a major effort for my wife. Next came a back and forth motion. After each effort there was a minute or two of rest. The therapist cautioned us that Const should not do anything to tire herself, and we were again warned about using any force whatsoever on her arm.

While the therapist talked, I became aware that it was all directed at Const, as if I weren't there. This was to hold true throughout the many weeks of therapy at two hospitals; with only one or two exceptions, it was as if I did not exist. "Good morning, Connie," "Hello, Connie," "How are you, Connie?" While I was always welcome, I became the invisible man in therapy. This treatment was accorded all other "surplus" people, and my only critique of the wonderful job the therapists did was that they did not include the patient's caregiver in therapy sessions.

Sandwiched in between physical and occupational therapy was speech therapy. After several sessions, Candice, the speech therapist, gave Const a visual test on concentration, eyesight, and the thought process in general. She passed the test with flying colors. In fact, when she was tested on arithmetic, she was answering the questions faster than I was! It was a relief to know there were no problems in these areas.

After a half hour in occupational therapy, where hand and arm work were done, we'd move over to physical therapy where foot and leg manipulation were performed. The process of gently moving the affected part, during which the therapist talked to it all the while, became a way of life every morning and afternoon for the next two weeks. I could see progress being made and so could Const.

While there was little or no control of her hand, arm, and leg, she was gaining movement. It hurt to see her arm flailing uselessly in the air, out of control, but it indicated that eventually, with muscle tone, control would return. Only time would tell how much.

A positive attitude became the key to success. I had always known that it would play a part, but I never realized how vital it was. From watching other patients in therapy, I became convinced that a positive outlook was nearly everything in recovery. If the patient became discouraged easily, very little could be done for them, since they felt it was useless to cooperate. I felt for the patients who gave up on themselves, and after a few days I didn't see them around anymore. Some probably went home, and others most likely went to nursing homes. In order to make strides in recovering from a stroke, it seemed to me that you first must be absolutely committed to helping yourself.

In fairness to some patients, the damage they'd suffered may have been too great to hope for any dramatic recovery. But in many instances, patients seemed to give up on themselves when a little grit and determination might have made a world of difference. Const had enough of these qualities to spread some around to other patients and still have enough for herself.

During the first few days of therapy, Const confided to me that she hated it. Within a few days, though, she started to look forward to it as sort of a personal competition with herself. Needless to say, I welcomed this attitude.

After about a week, she was chatting with a new acquaintance down in therapy. This lady felt it was no use trying; she couldn't go through the therapy regime. Upon hearing this, Const looked up at the woman's husband, who shrugged helplessly.

Const tried to change the woman's attitude, even to the point of scolding her. "Do you want to spend the rest of your life in a wheelchair?" she asked.

In spite of Const's words, we did not see her in therapy for awhile, and assumed she had given up. Then one day she was back at the hospital, and Const wheeled up and greeted her warmly.

"I decided I didn't want to spend my life in a wheelchair," she said. "At least not if I could help it." Her husband put a hand on Const's shoulder, and with tears in his eyes, said "Thank you."

At the end of two weeks in the hospital, the doctor who was assigned to Const drew me aside and inquired as to whether I thought I could handle her at home. I had to give an honest answer, but thought that if she could not come home, she would be in a nursing home, at least temporarily. He informed me, however, that there were two other options. Although she was not quite ready for out-patient treatment, there were two facilities that specialized in care for stroke victims. One was in downtown Minneapolis, and the other was a hospital fairly close to our home. She would be hospitalized for an additional two weeks, then go for out-patient treatment as long as she showed signs of improvement. Although she'd made great strides since the onset of the stroke, I knew I could not handle her alone at home in her present condition.

While I knew of the downtown hospital and its excellent reputation, I chose the other facility for convenience. This in spite of the fact that the IRS would have allowed my driving expenses as a deduction—the only such health care related deduction we were qualified to receive.

Normally, Const and I discuss matters of any major importance. However, I did not discuss the options with her at this point. The doctor expected an immediate answer, and since both facilities were equally recommended, I gave him one.

Once the person is ready to leave the hospital, the next step in the recovery process depends on the degree of physical limitation and the potential for further rehabilitation. For some patients who have had a milder stroke, they may be able to return directly home. They may need an ambulation device such as a walker or a cane, and might require some modifications to the home. Throw rugs might be removed from the floors to help prevent the possibility of the person slipping on them, and the bathroom might be modified by putting a bar by the toilet, installing a raised toilet seat, or by purchasing a shower chair. The therapists at the hospital can make recommendations on what devices would be most helpful to the patient's unique situation and needs. If necessary, a home care therapist can go out to the home and evaluate it for safety.

When some individuals return home after a stroke, they may still have a need for some ongoing therapy. Therapy can be done on an out-patient basis or by having the therapist come to the home. The advantages of out-patient therapy is that the very acts of getting up, dressed, and out to therapy are essentially acts of therapy themselves. Out-patient therapy can generally be done five times a week, or whatever is recommended by the primary physician.

Home therapy may be needed for the individual who is unable to go out. Most often, home therapy is done three times per week, but it may be more or less often, depending on the physician's recommendation. If the stroke survivor has additional needs, home health care can be arranged to meet them. A home care nurse can draw blood if necessary and can monitor the person's vital signs and medications. A home health aid can assists with bathing and physical cares as needed.

In order for Medicare or most insurances to pay for home care, the person must be "homebound." If the individual is physically able to come to the hospital for therapy, he or she won't qualify for coverage of expenses for home services. Even when a stroke survivor is confined to the home, Medicare and private insurance company coverage is generally fairly minimal. The person may be eligible for a limited number of health care visits for a certain number of weeks after hospitalization.

If additional home care is necessary, extended hours can be arranged for three to twenty-four hours a day, but this is a service that the individual will have to pay for privately. The stroke survivor and the family should check with their social worker about the programs available in their area. There are a variety of community resources that are often available to help the person remain independent in their home. Some of them are: meals on wheels, chore and cleaning services, shopping services, transportation, social and recreational programs, and emergency response systems. In this last service, the individual wears a pendant with a button on it around the neck, and pushes it when in trouble. It rings the area hospital's emergency room. The social worker can help the stroke survivor and family gain information on and access to such programs.

Mary, the social worker, asked Const if she wanted to transfer to the other hospital by ambulance, by medicab, or by our private vehicle. Of course, she opted for our station wagon. We were to report in at 2:30 that afternoon at the rehab center. It was only 1:30 when we left, and the other hospital was not that far away.

Now it so happens an ice cream parlor with the best ice cream in the world was in the opposite direction on this pleasantly warm early May afternoon. Feeling like a couple of teenagers out for a lark, we decided the hospital could wait while we enjoyed a couple of double dips. I knew that Const could use a little R and R after two weeks of trauma.

"We expected you an hour ago," were the first words out of the receptionist's mouth when we finally reported. Like a couple of guilty children we smiled and apologized for being late. Our whereabouts remained our secret.

This new hospital was much larger and more complex than the other one. We were escorted to the top floor and informed it was reserved exclusively for rehabilitation patients.

Our first surprise was the room. It was of normal size, but it contained only one bed. As we were to discover, each of the rooms had just the one bed, unlike other floors in most hospitals. There was a reason for it, we were to learn.

"Dinner is served in the main dining room," the nurse informed us. "Unless you have a very good reason, you will eat with the others." She told us Const would walk to dinner. Holy smoke! Const would be glad to walk there on her hands pushing a peanut with her nose, if only she could. If they could get her walking, we were all for it, but then the nurse corrected herself, explaining that she meant they wanted Const to go down to dinner in her wheelchair rather than eat in her room.

She showed us around the room briefly. The fact that there were two closets indicated it had originally been an average hospital room, occupied by more than one patient at a time. We had a nice view of a golf course, and the nightstand came equipped with all the necessities.

But would my insurance company pay for the private room? I asked the nurse and she told me they would.

Like many decisions, a person may not appreciate the importance of a choice made on an insurance plan at the time it is made. I thanked my lucky stars we had decided on our present coverage. While the premiums seemed excessive, I had seen the bill for Const's anuerysm hospitalization, and it could have choked a moose. Private rooms like the one she was in now were certainly more costly than her double room had been, although I didn't know how much more.

While most of us realize how important it is to have proper health care, many people look at health insurance as if it were a craps game at a casino. They want to "play the odds" that they will remain healthy. Unfortunately, none of us is immune from the possibility that we could develop an illness that could have long term effects and run up large medical expenses. For this reason, it is a good idea to evaluate health care insurance coverage on an annual basis.

It has become impossible to choose one type of insurance and be assured that it will always be the very best one for your needs. In evaluating different plans and insurers, the consumer should compare a plan with others on the market in terms of cost and deductibles, coverage, and extra services that may be included.

For example, a person can find out if the insurance company only contracts with certain facilities for rehabilitation and nursing care, if in fact these services are covered at all in the plan. The consumer should also weigh the advantages and disadvantages of an HMO versus a private insurance company. A very common misconception that Medicare recipients have about their HMOs is that they are a supplement to Medicare. They believe that if the HMO doesn't pay, they can use Medicare. What they don't understand is that by signing up for an HMO while under Medicare, they have transferred the Medicare benefits over to the HMO.

It's always helpful to be up to date in your knowl-

edge of your health care benefits. No one wants to be surprised by an increase in insurance rates after a devastating illness has occurred.

From the nurse's manner, I was beginning to wonder if this was a military hospital, but then she smiled at Const and said, "Welcome. Your stay here will depend on you. We expect you to do as much for yourself as you can. A therapist will be up at seven in the morning to help you dress. We will do everything we can to get you back to normal, but it all depends on you."

At about five-thirty that evening, patients in wheelchairs, some with canes and some supported by one or two aids or nurses, began to converge on the dining hall. They were all going down to dinner in the best way they were able. The queen rode her black chariot into the dining room with her one horsepower husband carefully negotiating around various obstacles.

The evening meal was a new experience. Nurses, aids and family all pitched in to cut meat, butter bread, and otherwise assist each patient. The dining room was large, but it was still difficult to manuever among the tables and wheelchairs.

This meal gave both Const and I a sense of perspective. While any stroke is a horrible experience, we learned there were other people who had it a lot worse than Const did. Some of them were relatively helpless, and cried when they tried to speak. Others laughed uproariously for no reason. Some could walk beautifully, but had lost the use of a hand, arm, or their ability to speak.

No two strokes are identical. This is because everything depends on the location of the damage to the brain. The problem can occur anywhere, which accounts for the drastic differences in the patients. The doctor told me that Const's damage was deep inside the brain, yet it did not affect her speech.

By the time dessert was served, the room was beginning to buzz with social noises. Const had already decided she liked two of the people at her table, but the third would be avoided in the future. This woman had an overbearing manner and was very demanding of the nurses, aids, and visitors who were helping to prepare the plates. After many years of marriage, I was able to detect Const's little signs, and knew she wanted to steer clear of this patient whenever possible.

We have a secret signal system just between the two of us to convey our emotions in the presence of other people. Three little squeezes with the hand means "I love you," and four in return is the reply, "I love you, too." Over the years we have developed other squeeze signals to convey our secret feelings in public. At times it seems like Morse Code flying silently between us. In this instance she reached over and touched my arm, and squeezed twice while flashing her eyes in the direction of the offending dinner guest. Two squeezes is about the bottom of the ladder in personalities. I blinked my eyes twice in rapid succession in response; I agreed with her assessment.

Over the years I have revealed this secret communication method to a few couples, and the most rewarding result came from one whose marriage had been on the rocks. They told us the "love code" had saved their relationship more than once since we confided in them. It seems that after a spat, neither of them would voice an apology, but they found that three little squeezes did the trick.

The morning following our arrival at the new hospital, a therapist arrived right on schedule to prepare Const to go downstairs only to find she had already dressed herself. Her ingenuity had certainly not been damaged by the stroke, and the nursing staff and therapist were duly impressed. Const told anyone and everyone, "I'm going to make it." The grim look of determination on her face as she did exercises, and the exhalation of breath as she completed a task told the story—she would succeed against all odds.

The next morning Const was down at the dining hall for breakfast by seven, and by seven-thirty was on her way to therapy. Therapy was conducted on a much larger scale than at the other hospital. I was astounded by the array of tools and gadgets and makeshift devices used to tone and strengthen the muscles. There was even a staircase that went up four steps and then down again; there was no challenge found in the home that wouldn't be addressed here.

It was beginning to dawn on me that the purpose of therapy was as much to recover as many of the skills required for normal activities as possible as it was to regain as much of the normal use of the body as the patient had previously. For example, we learned that Const would be taught how to peel a potato using only one hand, and how to bake a cake. The reason for assigning only one person to each room was to help promote the patient's sense of independence.

One hour of gentle workouts in physical therapy was followed by one hour of speech therapy and then one hour of occupational therapy. The usual approach during these sessions would be five minutes of exercise and then five of rest. This rigorous routine of three separate hours of therapy was repeated in the afternoon.

For the first few days Const dreaded and hated therapy at the new hospital, but then she began to look forward to it. Her progress was no doubt part of the reason for her change of heart. Also, she enjoys getting to know new people, and I think perhaps she was warming up to the new batch of therapists.

Over the weeks she became a big favorite of all them. Everyone knew her name, and even while busy with their own patients, they would look up, smile, nod and say hello.

Const made just as favorable impression on the nurses, and they treated her like royalty at all times. One night the queen mentioned to one of them that she wished she could have a bath. This was at eleven at night, and it was a rule that there were to be no baths after five p.m. Our daughter Barb was there, and the nurse looked at Barb and Barb looked at the nurse, and the same thought hit them both: why not?

"I'll get fired if they find out about this," the nurse said.

"I'll take responsibility," Barb replied. "If anyone comes by, you just say you were stopping me." The nurse agreed to the plan, and I'm glad that she would not let an administrative edict get in the way of a patient's well being.

"Let's go," the nurse said, packing Const into the wheelchair. She, Barb, and Const raced down the hall and into the bathroom, all three of them laughing hysterically as they pulled off their caper in the dead of night without anyone being the wiser. Talk about therapy! There's nothing like swiping a bath in spite of the rules and regulations to give a patient's morale a boost. Const had a sparkle in her eyes as she told me all about it the next morning.

My days became doubly busy. This hospital, while closer than the one downtown, was twice as far away as the first one where Const had been treated, and the only blessing was that most of it was freeway driving. I spent every day from about seven in the morning until nine at night with her and arrived home too tired to worry much about dinner. Sam, our huge black cat, and Missy, our German Shepherd, would demand my immediate attention. Both would be waiting at the door when I arrived home long after dark.

The demands on me were lightened a little when the hospital staff suggested I arrive at the hospital a little later in the morning, when Const's therapy began. The schedule still wore me down, but at six feet and two hundred pounds, I could well afford to wear down a little.

I didn't do too much cooking during this time, but when even the best greasy spoons began to get to me, I planned some simple meals. Full course dinners could wait until Const got home.

After two weeks of hospital care and therapy,

Const could begin to think about going home. A couple of hurdles remained, however. First, she was given an overnight pass.

That evening was the first time that three of our grandchildren (our daughter Barb's kids) saw Const since the "accident." Kathi, our oldest grandchild, ran into the bathroom crying when she saw her grandmother. At ten, she had the greatest understanding of what had happened. Eric, at three, simply said "Hi" and went off to look for some of the toys we kept for him. Karen, who had just turned seven, studied Grandma for a moment and then, stepping close, very carefully lifted Const's helpless left arm and placed it around her own shoulders. She said, "I still love you, Grandma."

Family members may attend therapy sessions to educate themselves on the techniques while learning the patient's strengths and limitations. When they visit the patient outside of therapy, they will then be able to encourage the individual to practice some of the tasks independently.

The most important function of family and friends, however, is to serve as the patient's "cheerleaders," to help keep the patient motivated, positive, and encouraged. It is natural for them to feel sorry for their loved one and want to help out with various tasks, but this may actually hinder rather than help recovery, as too much assistance can create frustration and dependency on the part of the patient. Instead, family and friends should applaud their loved one's achievements and encourage independence.

Health crises seem to bring out the very best and the very worst in people. While some family and friends may be very supportive and helpful, others may want to stay away from the patient. It might seem like they think stroke is contagious, but often when people don't know what to do or say, they choose to do nothing. Also, they may be uncomfortable because the stroke that their loved one experienced has forced them to consider their own mortality and realize how fragile life really is.

It's important to keep children and grandchildren involved with the stroke survivor. Before visiting, the parent should explain to the child what has happened in simple language she will understand. The different medical devices that the patient may be using should also be explained. The child should be allowed to ask questions and should determine the length of the visit and how close to get to the stroke survivor. Children tend to have an acute awareness of how the adult is feeling, and if the adult is anxious or fearful, they tend to react in the same way.

Since that first night went fairly well, Const was allowed to go home again for the following weekend. After each event, we were grilled on how it went.

The final test came in the hospital, on three successive evenings. Const would have to be on a blood thinning medication for the rest of her life, and it would be her responsibility to take a pill at six every evening for her last three days in the hospital. The pill would be put within easy reach at about four in the afternoon, and she would be checked at about six-thirty to see if she remembered to take it. I was told not to help her with this mental task while in the hospital; at home would be a different matter.

She passed the test with flying colors, but I wondered what would have happened if she hadn't. Would the hospital staff recommend sending her to a nursing home, keep her in the hospital longer, or send her home anyway and hope I would remember? Fortunately, she did remember, and to this day she seldom forgets.

The big day came and she was released, after spending a total of twenty-one days between the two hospitals. She had undergone two weeks of therapy in the second facility, four hours each day.

When the attendant wheeled her outside, she held up her hand to stop for a moment. "I just wanted to enjoy a breath of fresh air," she said, having lived with that disinfectant hospital smell for too long.

Oh, boy! Now, I thought, we could get back to a relatively normal routine and things would be easier for me, not having to chase to the hospital and cram the housework into my few spare moments. Of course, there would be several months of out-patient treatment, but I imagined that the new schedule of daily two hour visits would be a comparative relief.

How wrong I was. The fun was only beginning. Now that the queen of the hive was back in her domain, she was determined that things were going to get done on her schedule and in her way.

I didn't contradict her, but I prepared my own mental schedule, in which matters of a pressing nature were attended to first, and others were allowed to slide. My primary concern was to keep her spirits up and fill her day with things to keep her mind off the challenges she was facing.

Const enjoys good food, and I figured I would need to seek her advice on a variety of culinary matters. But when it came to laundry, I thought I already knew everything I needed: the washing had to be separated into whites and colors. I thought she was unnecessarily complicating things when she informed me that there were intermediate colors, too. Not if I could help it, there weren't.

She could not negotiate the basement steps to get down to our laundry room, so I was free to do things my own way at the washing machine. The first load of clothes that I brought up the stairs was intercepted by Wheelchair Connie and inspected. Traces of pink on some of the lighter colored clothes came from a guilty pair of red socks of mine.

I blamed the socks, but she was having none of it. "Try washing the clothes again in clean, cold water with lots of bleach." Rewashing did help somewhat, but I'd never had this problem before. It figured that something like this wouldn't happen until she got home.

As I labored at my duties, Const had her own schedule, not the least of which was the therapy to be performed at home. Most of it she could do on her own, but some of it did require my help. Her personal needs also required some assistance; it was particularly difficult for her to negotiate the tiled bathroom floor. I tried to help as much as I could without offending her.

Getting around the house in the wheelchair was manageable for Const, but by no means easy. Still, she kept on the go enough to thoroughly confuse me. After all, when she headed in the direction of the bathroom, I did not know if that was her intended destination or if she merely wanted to go to the kitchen for coffee. There were spots where she needed my help to move the wheelchair, and she would often set off without letting me know. If I did not read her mind and assist her, I would earn a cutting remark. Fortunately, this soon passed as she settled down emotionally and realized that being at home was not the same as it had been before her stroke.

However, my Const's fierce sense of independence and strong determination to get well carried over into our daily routine. I was willing to accept some direction around the house, so long as it fit my abilities and sensibilities. There were some things, however, that didn't go down well with me.

For example, moving every chair in the house when I vacuumed on the possible chance a speck of dust might be lurking there was hardly my style. To my mind, the middle of the rooms needed going over about once a month. Const and I reached grudging compromises on this and other chores.

Gradually, some organization began to evolve out of the messes I perpetually got myself into. If I could only have aligned my thinking and done my planning based on my her experiences, things would have gone more smoothly. Unfortunately, this is easier to talk about than to do. I was always used to making my own decisions and doing my own planning, and to suddenly listen to someone else's advice does not come easily to me.

I eventually discovered that if I could follow her advice and not make it appear I was doing so, it made both of us happy.

Reflections of an Occupational Therapist

by Constance S. Shaffer, OTR

Constance Saathoff Shaffer is the occupational therapist who first worked with Mrs. Collins after her stroke, and who continued to provide therapy throughout much of her recovery. In this piece she offers her perspective on Mrs. Collins' progress.

It had been a busy day in the hospital, and the referral on a new CVA, or cerebrovascular accident patient, was just one of many items on my schedule. I had enough time for a quick session to obtain some baseline data on the new patient, a Mrs. Constance Collins. (The baseline data describes what the patient can do on the first day of evaluation; all subsequent testing is compared to what is observed and recorded during this first session.)

Walking into Constance's room was like walking into The Spanish Inquisition. After the first five minutes, I knew this wasn't going to be brief. Constance was semi-reclined in bed, with family all around her.

"Hi," I began, "I'm Connie from Occupational Therapy. In case you're not familiar with what Occupational Therapy does, we work with people to help them get back to where they can be independent in taking care of themselves and resume their normal routines."

Shortly after my introduction, the questions started flying, most of them the kind that medical professionals can never answer definitively: "Will I get better?" "How long will it be until I get better?" "What should I be doing?"

I answered the questions as thoroughly as possible, throwing out all the statistics I had learned at school along with many of my experiences from my five years of working with CVA victims. I told Constance that the patient never gets one hundred percent recovery, but that it was my job to help her regain as much as possible.

"The sooner your left side shows some movement," I said, "the better the prognosis. Strokes often occur overnight, but recovery is relatively slow. You'll see the greatest amount of return in the first six weeks, with continued progress for six months. After that you may continue to see some improvement for up to one and a half to two years.

"Don't expect to have things return overnight. You will probably see improvement in your leg first, and then your arm. The muscle return usually starts in the bigger muscles close to your body, then works its way down your leg and arm. Your hand will probably be the last thing to come back."

While trying to satisfy her questions I worked with Constance's left arm to see what we had to work with. I could barely feel some light muscle contraction in the shoulder, but otherwise her arm was flaccid, like a wet noodle.

In conversation, Constance said she was left handed, which meant we would have to change hand dominance. She was oriented (could tell me the month, day, date, where she was and what had happened to her), and had no visual or mental deficits from the stroke. This was helpful, since good mental capabilities of attention and concentration make it easier to work on muscle retraining and reeducation.

Constance kept falling to her right, requiring verbal instructions to pull herself upright. As I helped her correct her balance, I told her that this was a common problem with stroke victims: when loss of function is on one side, that side of the face, throat, and body are affected as well as the arm and leg. I told her that one of the first things that Occupational Therapy and Physical Therapy would do would be to work on helping her keep her balance—this had to be attended to before she could walk or dress herself.

I asked Constance if she could lift her left arm. She promptly grabbed it with her right hand and raised it over her head. I laughed, and said, "That's what I call cheating. Now, can you do it without using your right hand?'

51

"No," she replied, "it's dead."

I corrected her immediately. "Never say it's dead! It may be sleeping, out to lunch or just not listening, but not dead! That's as bad as saying 'I can't.' What we need to do is wake it up and get it going again.

"When you have a stroke it kills off a part of your brain. That part doesn't come back to life. What we need to do is build new pathways.

"Think of your brain as a network of roads. Where your stroke occurred there's major construction, and you can't get through that way anymore. What you need to do is find a detour, a new route that will get you to the same destination."

Constance nodded understanding at my explanation. Then she looked down at her arm, slapped it and said, "Wake up!"

She next asked about what she should be doing to help get it moving quicker. I replied, "The best thing you can do at this point is handle it with care. Wherever you are, make sure you know where your left arm is. Keep it in front of you and try to keep the hand flat. Don't let it make a fist.

"Put a pillow under the arm so that you keep your hand elevated above your heart. Because of the stroke, your circulation isn't able to pump the fluid out like it should, so there's more chance of your hand becoming swollen. If that happens, the muscles will become sore and stiff.

"When you move, make sure you take your left arm with you. Don't let it get caught underneath you in bed or fall off the wheelchair into the spokes of the wheel. When anyone moves you in bed or in the chair, don't let them grab your arm—make them lift you from behind your shoulder along your shoulder blade. For some reason, a lot of people think that a weak arm makes for good leverage.

"At this point, your arm is somewhat like a baby's. The shoulder muscles are very weak and can't handle much stress. Pulling on your arm or rolling over on it can cause subluxation, which is a dislocation or separation of the shoulder from the socket. It could also cause tearing of the muscle."

After forty-five minutes of questions and preliminary testing I was ready to make my exit. "You'll be seeing me twice a day for about thirty minutes each session. Since the doctor wants you on bedrest for now, I'll come up to see you. In a couple of days you should be able to start coming downstairs to our clinic. The focus of our sessions will be to get you independent enough to take care of your personal needs and to get that arm working again."

I was ready to leave when the inevitable question came up. "What about walking?"

"A physical therapist will be up later today to begin working with your leg and getting you walking again," I said.

"How is Occupational Therapy different from Physical Therapy?"

"The easiest explanation is that physical therapy will teach you how to get where you're going while occupational therapy will teach you how to do what you want to do when you get there. There's some overlap between the two, but we work on the same things for different reasons. Physical therapy may work on your sitting balance because you need that before you can walk. Occupational therapy will work on it so that you don't fall over when you reach down to put your socks and shoes on. The physical and occupational therapists generally work closely together to plan the treatment sequence."

Just from this initial session with Constance, I got the impression that she was a hard worker. In the following two weeks, I would learn that if anything, I was underestimating her.

She was highly motivated, following through on everything that was requested of her and more. In fact, she was generally too hard on herself, and was always frustrated with what she considered slow progress.

Constance had what is called "emotional lability," which is common among stroke victims. "Lability" means that the patient either laughs or cries inappropriately and has little control over when it happens. Constance's problem was crying, which frustrated and embarrassed her. It was just another part of her that was temporarily out of her control, and once she knew why she was crying and that this was simply another symptom of the stroke, she was able to begin working on regaining the control of emotion and deal with it in a positive way.

I went to Constance's room the first two days before she was cleared to come to the hospital's therapy clinic. There was perceptible progress in the muscle return of her arm; muscle was beginning to contract and move on its own without conscious effort. Along with the muscle return, however, came increased muscle tone, and this made it harder for her to control her arm and make it do what she wanted.

Increased muscle tone causes the muscle to contract, remaining tight. When one muscle is tight, then the opposite muscle is unable to work against it. For example, you have one set of muscles that help you make a fist and one set of muscles that open your hand. If the ones that make a fist all have increased tone (increased tone is usually in a group of muscles rather than in just one muscle) and cause your hand to close, the muscles that open your hand have to relax to allow the other ones to work. This happens throughout your body with muscles which move your bones in alternate directions.

In the case of stroke victims, the muscles on one side all tighten so that the other ones can't work, which can lead to increased rigidity, painful joints and stiffness. This increase in tone is not a conscious action, but it is controlled by the brain. When the patient tries to work against it, the effort often just increases the tone further.

Our first task was to work on Constance's ability to bathe, dress and groom herself. She was aided by the fact that her balance improved rapidly, and before long she could move around and shift her weight in the wheelchair without listing sideways.

When taking these first steps, sponge bathing under supervision of a therapist is probably the hardest thing for a patient to do. In other cases, nurses perform the task and the patient is often a passive participant. When working with an occupational therapist, however, the patient must struggle through a procedure that may by itself cause embarassment, made worse by the fact that the therapist must stand by and critique the patient's efforts without providing much help. To teach someone how to wash their right arm when the left one doesn't work, or wash their buttocks when they can't stand alone can be a frustrating experience, to say the least.

Constance, however, never let inconvenience bother her and took every new task as a challenge which she knew she could conquer. She achieved independence in her bathing within two sessions and was refusing assistance from the nurses by the end of the week. The carrot at the end of the stick was the day they would let her try the shower.

Dressing was mastered just as quickly, with Constance overcoming the obstacles of putting on socks and buttoning blouses with one hand through determination and constant practice.

Constance's determined nature was both her best trait and her biggest drawback in therapy. On the positive side, it gave her the willpower to work through her disabilities and overcome obstacles. On the other hand, she was her own worst critic. She was unrelenting on herself, never accepting "good" as the best she could do at a given moment. She was always mad at herself for not having done better. No amount of encouragement from her therapists could make her see that her progress was satisfactory.

Her physical therapy was also going well. As her balance improved, they had her taking some steps in the parallel bars, and she soon advanced to a quad cane (named for the four prongs at its end). Constance was terrified of falling at first, but improved rapidly with encouragement and her usual persistence.

El, her devoted husband, was present at all therapy sessions unless Constance chased him away. He was her personal cheerleader and kept her motivation up by accepting what she could accomplish at any given time and supporting all her rehabilitation efforts.

On the ninth day of therapy, Constance greeted me by saying, "Connie, my fingers are moving!" She proceeded to show me how her fingers could close on an object. She was ecstatic and her face was beaming. An olympic athlete couldn't have matched her feeling of accomplishment. We had worked with her hand and arm twice a day since our first meeting, and here was what she had been waiting for—to see those fingers moving. It gave her hope that things might turn around, that there was a real chance for a thorough recovery.

At that time, therapy sessions consisted of bilateral exercises using Constance's right arm to guide and train the left with relearning movements, and passive motions in which I moved her arm. When movement began returning to it we worked on the skateboard, which looks very much like the toy you're probably familiar with. Constance's arm was strapped to its surface, allowing her to move it without the handicaps of gravity and friction. Vertical, horizontal and diagonal movements were soon mastered. It was quite a bit tougher to advance to lifting the arm off the table to grab a glass, and it would be quite a while before that feat could be accomplished. Constance often became depressed with her inability to perform the harder tasks, and required both encouragement from the therapists and some wonderful pep talks from El.

Constance was transferred out of my hospital to a rehabilitation center approximately two weeks after I first began working with her. She was nervous about leaving a now familiar and "safe" environment, but was eager to continue her rehabilitation.

I saw Constance and El several times after she was discharged from the rehabilitation center. El had started to attend the hospital rehabilitation stroke support group meetings while Constance was in the hospital, and they both continued to do so every month. Every time they came to the clinic to see me, Constance had a new story to tell me about her increasing independence and her ability to use her left hand and arm.

Four

A New Routine

Within a few days of Const returning home, we settled into a routine. Three days a week I would take her over to the hospital for outpatient treatment. There was a golf course across the street from the hospital, and the therapy sessions took about two hours, so I entertained the idea of passing the time out on the greens and fairways. However, when it came time to drive out to the hospital, I found that I did not have any desire to get in nine holes during those two hours. Someday I may add that course to the long list of golf courses I have played over the years, but I never took the opportunity during Const's therapy.

Besides my great concern for the health of my beloved, I must admit that I was fascinated by the capabilities and techniques used by the therapists. Objects of all kinds were utilized for therapy. Hula hoops, balls from the size of beach balls all the way down to golf balls, clothespins, and other items played significant parts. Each muscle had to be worked separately, from the largest leg muscle to the smallest muscle in the little finger. All of the gadgets and items were intended to aid in muscle exercise.

For the finger muscles, a putty not unlike nutty putty was used. The therapist pulls it out in a string and laces it around the affected fingers. (The feature that distinguished this stuff from nutty putty was that it was not at all sticky.) It took Const all the effort she could muster to force her fingers apart. In all likelihood, a six month old baby would have had no problem doing this.

To really strengthen any muscle, resistance has to be used, but unfortunately, a muscle that cannot freely move a leg or a finger is in no position to work against much resistance. It has to be motivated, without tiring the patient in the process. The putty was ideal for finger therapy; its tad of resistance was all Const's fingers could handle. The thickness increased gradually as the muscles responded over a period of weeks. The putty was sent home with her so she could practice at the kitchen table.

All the tools of the trade are used with the same purpose in mind, to create a small resistance for an afflicted muscle and work up in small increments. However, many of the items we saw were never incorporated into Const's workouts. The therapists were free to use whatever items they thought would be effective.

One of them suggested we buy a one-handed can opener, and showed me this ingenious tool. I spent an entire day trying to locate one with no luck; it seems the company that made them no longer produces this item. It was, however, a comical episode when a salesman tried to convince me he had a model that could be used with one hand. After he finished his spiel I asked him to put his hand in his pocket and show me how it worked. It didn't; the attempt only embarrassed him.

While I was intrigued by the gadgets and methods employed by the therapists, I was also impressed by their consistent cheerfulness and positive attitudes. A quiet confidence pervaded the atmosphere where they worked. They were all business as they tried to instill confidence in the patients, and although a lot of friendliness went into their efforts, there were no displays of sympathy. If the patient would not adopt the right attitude after several weeks, they were out. There were too many waiting for help to spend time on those who wouldn't help themselves.

In my view, willpower and determination are a big part of the battle. Therapy is not easy, and we were told right up front that most of the recovery would take place in the first six months, and that it could take three years or longer to get back as much of the normal usage as the "accident victim" would ever recover.

There was reason for hope, though. Const and I had seen stroke victims who enjoyed full lives with little or no limitations. I was first introduced to them at therapy meetings while Const was undergoing physical manipulation therapy during the first week after the stroke. She began to attend them with me after she had "graduated" from the second hospital and was in outpatient therapy.

Bonnie, a motherly type who had more years on the job than any of the other nurses, had informed me of my attendance in no uncertain terms on the fourth day in the hospital. "I'll come and get you at two p.m. this afternoon—I want you to attend a meeting." In a nice way she had told me I had no choice.

I can't speak for victims of other types of illnesses, such as cancer or heart attacks, but the stroke patient has support groups located right in the hospital and at public buildings supplied by city services. The groups build up a comraderie of support, and the person who does not take advantage of them is the big loser.

Bringing together "accident" patients periodically is a means of therapy not only for the victim, but for the caregiver and family members as well. The hour-long sessions usually begin with a speech of encouragement by someone in charge, followed by an open discussion on problem solving, the offering of suggestions, and the recounting of experiences. Or, the hour may be taken up by a guest speaker on any subject even remotely related to the victims. Topics include: where to get financial help, how to find persons willing to sit with the victim, how to conduct personal business, like shopping, and any other subject the group may find of interest.

The faces change at each meeting, but the routine usually stays the same. A very successful meeting ends with a victim getting up and prancing around the room. You can imagine the reaction of a patient upon seeing someone who was in the same boat as himself at one time show this kind of recovery! It's a real morale builder.

When Bonnie escorted me into a room full of people that first time, I could see that half of them were obviously stroke victims. After introductions all around, each of us told our sad story about an "accident" and how it had affected us. Amusing anecdotes and funny observations helped relieve the pressures.

The experience was eye-opening. I realized that I was walking around in a world of illusions, functioning normally, yet under pressures that made what was happening seem unreal and removed from my life. Const, a charming, loving person, had been knocked down without the slightest provocation or warning. When I saw her in the hospital bed, I could have broken down in sobs. But I wouldn't let myself do that, I couldn't show my emotions to her as she desperately clung to me for strength. I needed to show my unwavering support for her.

I could only guess what was going through her mind, but she never asked "Why me?" She didn't cry, at least not in front of me. That terrifying first day, she only complained that her face felt numb, as if a dentist had given her a shot of novocaine. She knew what had happened to her; after all, she had diagnosed it on the telephone with the doctor. I actually wanted her to have a good cry, because I was afraid that if she eventually did break down after holding back, it would be uncontrollable.

My increased responsibilities at home filled the day and sometimes the night as I struggled to give support and encouragement to Const while I provided taxi service, made meals, picked up the house, did the washing, some ironing, took care of the yard and garden, mowed the lawn, and attended to our pets, Sam and Missy.

I jokingly told people I had just discovered where the washing machine was. Of course, I had known where it was, but had refused to go near it other than to dig out a load of clothes when Const called down the clothes chute. I would either toss them in the dryer or bring them upstairs; that was the extent of my experience with the laundry. In those first days when my wife was hospitalized, I simply guessed at what I didn't know and kept my fingers crossed.

While Const was in the hospital, one of my best kept secrets was completely shattered. She had a favorite blouse which I washed for her while she was staying at the hospital, then recognized it needed ironing. I hauled out the ironing board from the broom closet and set it up, then found the iron in a lower cupboard stall near several spray bottles containing liquids of various colors. I plugged in the iron to let it heat while I sprayed the garment with one of the bottles.

Many years had passed since mother made me iron "just in case I might have to someday." Some small detail might be overlooked, I thought, but the job seemed to go along pretty well. Finishing my prize, I carefully folded it up and hurried to the hospital to present it to my cherished one.

The look on her face was one of dismay, followed by utter disbelief. I turned the article around to give it a closer inspection. It was loaded with wrinkles.

"It needs ironing," she stated flatly.

"I did iron it," I confessed.

"You couldn't have." She decided to test me. "Where do I keep the ironing board?"

"In the broom closet."

"That was a lucky guess," she said, as my frustration increased over the fact she did not believe me. "Where do I keep the iron?"

Now I was getting ticked—she was all but accusing me of lying! "In the first big cupboard beside the refrigerator along with the spray bottles," I replied.

Apparently she was beginning to believe me. "You must not have had enough heat on the iron. Was it on the cotton setting?"

"Yes," I lied. I remembered having glanced at the setting and figuring it was alright.

"Well then, you didn't have it plugged in!"

Now that was an insult I couldn't overlook. No one would be stupid enough not to plug it in. Maybe dumb enough not to see if it was heating, but not stupid enough to leave it unplugged.

"I can't wear it like that," she announced with finality.

I have seen times when I was glad to have anything to wear at all, much less worry about what it looked like, but I stuffed the blouse into my back pocket and sat down. My action was not lost on her; for now, the subject was closed.

The following day I appeared with the blouse draped on a hanger in all its full glory. Const was truly pleased to see the garment wrinkle free. She opened her mouth to praise me, but like Brutus, she had one more thought for her Caesar.

"Who did you get to iron this?"

"Is it alright?"

"Yes, it's beautiful."

"Well then, does it matter who did it?"

"No, I guess not."

Had she pushed the issue any further I might have invented some beautiful blonde on the next block. At the time, the issue had been settled, but knowing the queen, I realized even then that it was not over. She was going to find out one way or the other just who did the ironing.

The truth of the matter is that I had neglected to inspect the setting on the iron carefully, and the heat was way too low. I had ironed it myself on the correct setting the next night. I cherished the compliment she unknowingly paid me on my second effort, but when she got home and found I had learned my way around the task of ironing, however, my secret was out.

Looking back on that last sentence, perhaps I was too hasty in pronouncing that I had learned how to iron. There was still one subtlety that had escaped me, and I didn't learn about it until after the queen had returned home.

I was ironing a few items periodically, enough to keep my wife in her favorite blouses. It was a small enough chore, but I learned that it could lead to total destruction of the male ego.

Const kept all the secret weapons for housecleaning in a cupboard next to the refrigerator, and that was where I found the iron. Alongside of it was a bottle of water, which I assumed was used for spraying the garments about to be ironed in order to help induce the wrinkles to disappear. I had been spraying the clothes with this bottle of water for several months; after all, I knew better than to use one of the spray bottles with colored liquid in them—they're for washing windows and such.

My wife has a nose like a German Shepherd; our dog Missy could take lessons from her when it comes to tracking down strange scents. Each time she put on one of the blouses she would sniff it thoughtfully, but make no comment. Then one morning I got up early just to do some ironing, because she had told me she was going to try to do it herself. She wasn't ready to handle the iron, but I suppose she was tired of seeing her blouses draped over a chair in the kitchen.

My ironing done, I was about to return all the cleaning supplies to the cupboard when I heard a shriek behind me.

"What have you been using to spray my blouses?"

"That bottle with water in it," I replied.

"That's ammonia water in there, not tap water!"

So that was why Sam and Missy went into such antics when they were accidentally sprayed. Sam would spend an hour washing himself, over and above his normal scrubbing time. I vowed to be more careful about what and where I sprayed. Sam and Missy deserved better.

One laundry related chore I thought would be easy was gathering up the dirty laundry. Even that proved to be a challenge, however, since I could not remember the kitchen hand and dish towels. They seemed to run and hide when I gathered up the wash.

If I didn't make an extra effort to remind myself they could become strong enough to walk to the basement by themselves.

As I've mentioned, when Const went to the hospital I was also given the job of making meals, a chore I continued when she came home, since she was still unable to stand. At first, canned goods frequently caught my attention when the frozen stuff gave out. Then there were the frequent trips to collaborate with the Colonel and to that terrific Chinese place not too far away.

Naturally, our food bill went up, so I began to venture into the kitchen more often. Then I began to notice that while the bills were going down, my weight was going up. I was not burning as many ounces as I was piling on. I finally discovered there was a reason other than my not shutting my mouth soon enough.

When I did venture into the kitchen, I could fry eggs and bacon and open a can of soup with the great chefs of the world. As I began to attempt more exotic dishes, however, I had to sample them as they progressed towards their culinary sublimity. It was necessary to test the potatoes to be certain they were done so they didn't end up looking like a hand grenade had exploded in the pot. There had to be a better way than stabbing them with a fork every two minutes. I realized I would have to go easier on the sampling. How had Const managed to make such excellent meals and still stay thin?

As I became more sure of myself in the kitchen, I began a practice that was responsible for some minor friction between the queen and her drone. While I knew what spices Const would use to season her dishes, I couldn't help wondering how they would taste with certain substitutes. For instance, I would try cider vinegar instead of white vinegar, and she would catch me at it and voice her disapproval. So the next time I'd secretly drop in a little lemon juice just to fix her wagon.

Sometimes she would compliment the meal, at least until she learned how I made it. Then she would never admit that it had come out tasting pretty good. I think I can say objectively that my cooking became tasty and nourishing; to support this statement, I'll modestly mention that Const put on an additional thirty pounds at one point. I thought she looked like a million bucks, but she didn't agree and started dieting.

I'll share some of my cooking secrets in a later chapter.

One chore I was already accustomed to was taking out the garbage, since I had been trained never to go outside for any reason without checking the bag. It had gotten to the point where I could feel her eyes boring into my back whenever I approached the back door.

Since hauling the garbage out was second nature, I thought that installing a new bag was something I could do alone without too much supervision. One inch of the bag had to be folded down to stabilize it and to allow the bag to be closed when full. No big deal. But now comes the Ann Landers part.

For weeks, people across the country wrote in to

her arguing about whether the toilet paper should unwind from the wall side or the outside of the roll. (For the record, we unwind from the outside when I install it, and from the wall side when Const does.)

In a similar manner, we have not resolved whether the saved grocery bags designated for future use as garbage bags should be placed in the container in the cupboard with the open end up or down. My wife contends that if the open end is down they will come out easier when removed. I feel they're harder to get in this way. I would shove them in sideways unless Wheelchair Connie arrived on the scene. When time permits, perhaps I'll take up the garbage bag problem with Ann.

I have by no means aired all of our dirty laundry, nor do I intend to do so. One of the underlying principles of rehabilitation is to try to maintain humor in the relationship. On the other hand, the victim can break down in tears over a piece of well intended humor. The caregiver has to understand these foibles. Being struck down without warning takes a dreadful toll on a person, and the physical disability is only part of the trauma. While free of any mental damage, Const's entire system needed restoring, and this included her sense of humor. I could only hope this was merely a temporary disruption, because her humor served us both well before the stroke.

For her part, she has always insisted that I have no sense of humor. My standard reply is "I married you, didn't I?"

Five

The Wheelchair Commando

Wheelchair Connie, the mechanized commando, had struck again. Too much vigor and not enough skill has caused her to topple her favorite plant (and vase) from atop a table where it had resided for many years. Travelling backwards in a wheelchair with nothing to guide you on the tight turns except your peripheral vision is a skill pretty much impossible to master, although she labored at it with all the determination of a six-year-old.

Our carpeting still has ruts in it which I doubt will ever come out. Most of the furniture is marred and scratched from hasty judgement, yet I am thankful that her eyesight is apparently undamaged. Some stroke victims will have a completely blind area where as much as a half a page in a book will seem not to exist. A person can be standing right next to them and they will not see half of that person's face.

In spite of the unintentional damage it has caused, however, the wheelchair served a useful purpose. It allowed Const to scoot into the darker recesses of a room and ferret out dust kitties and globs of dog hair which, if left to me, would remain untouched. When she found something she couldn't reach, nothing else would do except that I verify the condition and promise to clean it. Because I'd probably forget it otherwise, I found it best to drop whatever I was struggling with and clean up the problem immediately. That dog of ours has always been more trouble than it's worth, but Const loves it. Missy is a German Shepherd with a doubtful heritage.

The dog is hers. Sam, the sixteen pound black cat, is mine. Sam also sheds, but it doesn't show as much. There has always been one small problem between Const and me and Sam and Missy. Missy thinks I belong to her and Sam believes Const is his. This is something I'd never correct in the animals even if I could. The problem existed long before Sam arrived on the scene. I made the mistake of taking Missy for a ride in the back of my pickup, and she's been attached to me ever since. Now I can't make a move without her at my heels. And Sam gets very upset if Missy and I leave him behind. He also loves to ride, which is very unusual for a cat.

In Const's family, only dogs were allowed. In my family, any animal from a donkey to a gopher was acceptable as a pet. Prior to our getting serious about marriage, we covered the subject of pets in our future household.

"We can have dogs, but no cats," Const declared. She is of German descent, and can state her demands pretty forcefully. This was law.

However, having some English blood in me and remembering the battle of Britain, I replied, "No cats, then no dogs." I was never able to stick to this position, however. Through the many years of our marriage, we have almost always had a dog, and I inevitably wound up taking care of it. But we had no cats.

Then one day a friend casually mentioned she had seen a litter of kittens, and described how sweet and cuddly they were. A week later she mentioned them again, and this time she said one was all black.

I had always wanted a black cat, so I drew her aside and told her I would take it. Several days later she arrived with the kitten all wrapped up in a blanket, and brought along a complete care kit, including litter and a pan.

Const was speechless, but then surprise is good for any marriage. I knew she was a good sport, and that she knew fair was fair—I had threatened to get a cat every time a new dog had entered our house. Also, I was certain she could not resist a kitten as charming as this one, and I was right.

I named our new kitten Sam, aware that animals understand and respond better to short names. Const had decided on Missy, and it had taken hours to come up a name she approved of, so I avoided this happening again by quickly establishing our new pet's name myself.

Const silently watched as I made more of a display

over Sam than was really necessary. Her first introduction to the way of cats came when I poured the litter into the pan and dropped tiny Sam on top of it. She looked inquiringly at me as I turned and walked away.

"Sam is now housebroken," I stated simply. I privately hoped he would not make any mistakes. He did not. As he grew older and was able to climb the steps, I moved his pan to the basement. Const was pleased about the move, and to her credit, fully accepted Sam into the family.

While dogs are dumb enough to like people, cats reserve their right to call the shots from minute to minute. Sam thought Const's wheelchair was his private domain whenever it was unoccupied. This created some tension, since Const was unable to move him out of it with only one hand. Sam had no intention of giving up without being forced to, so I was called on to do the job.

There was another problem with Sam that still persists today. When he moves about, there is no sound of tramping feet as there is with Missy. Const and I have to know his whereabouts whenever we move around the house. She would be in serious trouble if she stumbled over him. But since he was always waiting to occupy the wheelchair the moment Const left it, the problem was actually minimized.

Const has learned to like Sam, although she won't show it, much less admit it. Yet Sam loves her and only tolerates me.

As a condition of keeping Sam, I had to assure Const that he wouldn't climb on the cupboards. I told her I could train him to stay off them. Unfortunately, there is no way I've found to train a cat not to climb. The instinct must have been in their genes since shortly after the big bang.

When Sam reached puberty, he was big enough to climb on the cupboards. Since Const likes to sleep later in the morning than I do, I would make sure that he was off of them before she got up. Then one day she confronted me.

"I thought you said you'd train that cat to stay off my cupboards."

"He is trained," I bluffed, wondering how she knew otherwise.

"Look." She stooped and pointed. "They're all over the place."

The little cat tracks looked just like the ones Sam left on the windshield and all over my truck's hood. There was no way to blame Missy for this. "I'll retrain him," I told her, hoping she'd buy it.

The next morning I washed all traces of Sam from the kitchen cupboards. The first thing Const did after getting up was to check out all the surfaces, but she didn't find the telltale marks. This went on for a week, until one morning when I was busily wiping up Sam tracks with my back turned to the bedroom door. I had forgotten to close it, and I heard a slight noise, like the clearing of someone's throat. Caught red-handed, I tried to explain that cats don't train all that well.

"Neither do husbands," was her reply.

The fact that Sam was always underfoot didn't exactly endear him to my bride, but he got the worst of it on at least one occasion, when he had his paw run over by the wheelchair. He fussed about it for a good five minutes, but it was his own fault for sticking close to Const in order to hop into her chair whenever she got up. The only time he left his post was when he got the opportunity to accompany me downstairs to the basement on a laundry run.

On one such occasion, I pulled the clothes out of the washer and stuffed them into the dryer before remembering to clean the lint filter. Pulling it from the inside back of the machine, I took it over to the garbage can by my workbench to empty it. I swung the dryer door out of the way as I left the area, leaving it ajar. When I returned, I could see a black tail protruding from the machine.

If it hadn't been for that waving tail, we would have had baked cat on our hands. I opened the door and Sam just stood there blinking, in no hurry to get out. Chasing him out, I thought that it was a good thing Const hadn't been there to see what he'd done. I didn't realize, however, that the incident wasn't over.

"Why does this towel have black cat hair all over it?" the inspector general demanded when I brought the laundry up.

Cats have fur, not hair, but I figured this bit of trivia wouldn't answer her question. I had to confess that Sam had almost gotten dried along with the clothes. To my surprise, Const scooped him up and hugged him.

If I have learned anything at all about women, it's that they're a lot smarter than men give them credit for. In fact, they're generally smarter than men. We educate engineers and pay them well to design products for use around the house. If enough complaints about the product motivate the company to look into a problem, they will invariably scout around for someone with a Ph.D. to help resolve the difficulty. Then that person rapidly becomes part of the problem because he has not soaked his hands in dirty dish water or had to launder clothes nearly enough times.

You would think they would ask the people who use these gadgets, but they've never solicited advice from Const after she's complained about the the stupid things she's found designed into our automatic clothes washer, or informed them that the combination screen and storm windows are backwards from what they should be. I've heard that some companies are beginning to listen to people who actually use their products. The right company could make a fortune by hiring Const as a consultant.

My bride is not only just as beautiful as the day we were married, but she is even smarter and more sophisticated. I have never seen a woman who can hold a candle to her. The trouble is, I can't get away with too much foolishness before she puts her finger on it, and no amount of bluster and conning will distract her. It is a good day when I can outfox Wheelchair Connie.

Still, I am dumb enough to believe that she thinks I'm pretty smart. I can also be dumb enough to think I'm smarter than she is. Somehow I forget that I'm the one who gets out there in the winter and shovels all the snow while freezing my buns off. I come in and she has hot chocolate, a kind word, and a pat on the arm, and I'm ready to go charging out to do battle with the elements again. I struggle in the chickweeds with the lawnmower, the sweat rolling off me, and she greets me with a cool lemonade which she has prepared while watching me from the air conditioned house to make certain I get in close enough to the shrubs. Of course, I realize that Const has always done her own share of work around the house, yet I'm still impressed with how she can not only see to it that I do mine, but also make me like it.

She has also been ingenious in devising tools to help her perform difficult tasks. For instance, she discovered that by wetting a dishrag she could twist it around the cap of the catsup bottle and pull it off.

The only tools I kept away from her after her stroke were the butcher and paring knives. Her medication keeps her blood thinned out, and a simple cut could have caused problems. So long as I was the one to peel the potatoes and slice the onions, this posed no difficulty, except when the thickness of the potato peelings came under her scrutiny. I took off too much skin, she said, but I got the eyes at the same time. She claims that much of the nutritional value of a spud is right next to the skin. For awhile my patience was right next to the skin as well.

Fortunately, any such annoyance was more than compensated for by the progress I saw in Const those first weeks. Even the smallest thing was an occasion for joy. It was a red letter day, for instance, when she was first able to hold onto a dish towel with her left hand. This may not seem like much unless you have been where we have. Every little success on her part was cause for rejoicing and celebration. Holding a railing, she learned to struggle up steps one at a time. Now and then we would take off her leg brace and try walking. To keep her foot from flapping out of control, we discovered that an Ace bandage wrapped around the knee, leaving the kneecap open, was a help.

Const hated that brace with a passion. Despite being plastic, it felt heavy to her and inhibited the use of her ankle. It was also difficult to get on and off, and could become uncomfortably warm.

After a number of small breakthroughs, I felt we had made a major one when I convinced her to take a shot at grocery shopping with me. It took a lot of talking to get her to agree, but I knew that it was important to get her back to normal routines as soon as possible, whether she liked it or not. Const had something which approached paranoia when it came to being seen with the chair, braces and an arm sling. I could sympathize with her, but I felt strongly about getting back into normal everyday business, even though the last thing I looked forward to was trying to manage a wheelchair and a grocery cart in a crowded store. The store where we shop is large and always seems to be busy.

Her major concern about going to the supermarket was that people would stare at her. I could understand this, but when I pointed out to her that handicapped people are all over the place, she agreed to try it. I did my best to keep her mind on shopping, but her interest in the vegetable department quickly waned and she disappeared towards the ice cream. The hard floors increased her chair speed tremendously, and I could see a smile flicker over her face as she roared down the aisles. A near collision with another wheelchair prompted a ten minute conversation with an auto accident victim.

She was beginning to recover some of the old verve for which she is locally famous. She quickly found two more people in wheelchairs to talk with, and I made up my mind to teach her semaphore so I could keep on shopping and make sure she knew where I was headed. I had all I could handle keeping track of her, but it was great to see her extroverted side come out once again.

It may be overwhelming for the individual to look at how they are today and then consider how far they hope to progress through therapy. The stroke survivor must form small, measurable and achievable goals rather than emphasize "the big picture." When the person starts to feel discouraged, as if he or she has taken two steps backward for every step forward, the individual can be reminded through the support of family and therapists of all that has been accomplished.

The use of humor can be helpful in therapy. It can release tension and help the stroke survivor develop a sense of perspective. Regaining the ability to laugh and joke is an important step in recovery.

The stroke survivor may feel self conscious about how he or she looks or communicates. Talking to others who have been through similar struggles can be very therapeutic for the stroke survivor. By sharing fears and concerns with someone who has been there, an individual can be given new hope that there is a full life to be had after a stroke. Peer counselor programs are available in many hospitals, and there are often stroke support groups in the community.

The other advantage of having Const accompany me to the supermarket was that I could benefit from her knowledge. One day I picked out about a half dozen peaches and brought them back to the cart. I went on to get something else, and when I returned, I saw that Const had removed them from the basket and was dumping them back in the bin.

"What's the matter?" I demanded, even though I knew that the peaches I selected often looked like thinly disguised baseballs. These small, round objects could easily be hit out of Wrigley Field without squashing them.

"These things will wither before they get ripe," she replied, sorting through the bin. "Pick up the peach like this," she instructed, holding a peach with her thumb near the stem area, "and push down gently on it. If the peach is anywhere near ripe it will be soft around the top."

I wished I'd known that all along; I could have saved some money. The grocer might stop ordering baseballs if all the shoppers knew this little trick.

***

The thought has occurred to me that this light-hearted approach is not in keeping with the harsh reality of the situation we faced every day. However, if I had not approached the problems in this manner back when the situation was at its worst, I might have broken down and cried when I looked at Const. This beautiful person, loved and admired by so many, had been struck down overnight by a vicious malady and temporarily turned into a near vegetable. She was, despite this, fortunate. Half of all stroke victims die, and many of the rest are left with some form of debilitating problem more severe than what Const has had to deal with.

By counting our blessings and keeping a healthy sense of humor, we were able to make it through the toughest times of those early days.

Six
My Little Red Truck

A few days after Const had her stroke, I decided to seek a way to take her mind off the catastrophe. She knew that my old pickup truck, which I used to enjoy driving, was giving me fits. I'd gotten used to the manual steering somewhat, but it needed new tires, a tuneup, and had a cracked windshield. It did have a sunroof of sorts—the roof leaked, in spite of all my attempts to fix it. This wouldn't have disturbed me except that the leak was right over the driver's side, so in cold wet weather I'd get ice water dripping down my neck. Of course, the truck was ideal for leaving in a parking lot; careless people could bash into it with their doors all they wanted and I wouldn't mind.

I began to tease Const about buying a new pickup, hoping to create a small difference of opinion to keep her zest and pluck engaged. From all the hints I dropped, I wondered if she thought that I'd already bought one and had it in the garage at home. My thinking was that if I could get her to worry more about what I was up to while away from her side, she wouldn't worry so much about herself. When at last I brought her home from the hospital, I watched her face as I opened the garage doors. As near as I could tell, I hadn't pulled her leg at all—she was not surprised at the absence of a new truck.

However, I kept up the charade as we drove to and from the hospital for outpatient therapy. I would point out red pickups to her whenever I spotted one.

"There's one!" I'd exclaim.

"One what?" she would inquire, feigning igno-rance.

"Right there! Isn't it a beaut?"

After several weeks of this, she began spotting red pickups herself, figuring that two could play at this silly game as well as one. So I had to take a new tack, pleased that she was fighting back. "No, that's the wrong brand," I would snort, or "That one's too big," or "That's Japanese—I want one that's made in the U.S." These replies never discouraged her, but rather prompted her to point out more red pickups. My plan was working; she was taking an active interest in my phony search.

One day on the way home from therapy, she said, "Why don't you check out that lot?" She pointed to a new car dealership.

I should point out that while it took twenty-five minutes to drive to the hospital, it generally took two to three hours to drive home, because Const enjoyed looking at houses. I didn't mind chauffeuring her around, though; anything to keep me away from housework. On this day Const had wanted to explore a new route, so we were in an area which was unfamiliar to me.

I almost spun our station wagon around, I turned into the truck lot so quickly. Not being seven kinds of a fool, I didn't need much of an opening. While I went out and kicked tires, she sat quietly in the car and observed her child trying to make up his mind which new toy to get.

My new truck didn't have to be red—that was simply part of my scheme to help keep her mind off herself. It did have to have power steering, though; the old one was sheer torture to maneuver into a tight spot. (I had no steering problems with it once it attained a speed of five miles per hour, but any turn at a lower speed than that was a killer.) I happened to find one that met all of my specifications, and it even happened to be red!

Now came the tough part, where Const would come into play. "She's going to fight this," I told the dealer. "She doesn't like the old one and she won't like the price, so you had better get your pencil sharpened real quick."

I'll leave you to guess which of them won the battle over the price—I just stood there trying not to be too impatient while they dickered. I do take care of balancing the checkbook, but Const makes the smart financial deals once I let it be known where I stand on an issue. If a product is a piece of junk, I don't hesitate to let the salesman know it. However, this little red truck was alright in my book, and at times I thought maybe Const was driving too hard a bargain. It was beautiful, but so was she!

As the deal was clinched and we left the lot, she said, "Now I would just as soon not hear any more about little red trucks." She smiled as she said it. Keeping me happy was still a goal in her life, despite her "accident."

Once again I had renewed appreciation for Const. Even after the long bout of haggling, the salesman insisted on filling the tank with gas—she had captivated him with her charm and manners. I always said she could charm the skin off a snake, and in all probability, the snake would thank her for it.

During the intervening weeks between initiating my scheme and actually buying the truck, Const's own personal method of transportation had improved, and this did a great deal to lift her spirits. When she was carted down to therapy by wheelchair that first week after her stroke, she said nothing, but I had the distinct feeling the wheelchair impressed upon her the debilitating nature of her problem. I knew she would feel much better when she was no longer so dependent on it.

I would be glad to get rid of it too, and at least a few of my reasons were entirely selfish. The chair was always in the way, and if our cat Sam wasn't in it or under it, our dog Missy was getting her tail stuck in the spokes. And even though the chair was a lightweight model, it took a heavy toll on my back. I could lift the chair in and out of our station wagon with no problem; it was the effort required to toss it far enough inside to close the tailgate that caused my back fatigue.

Unfortunately, my pickup truck was no solution, since Const could not climb into it. I would have to lift her in and out of it, and that would have only compounded my back trouble.

The problem was partially resolved when I discovered that the hospital had a bunch of wheelchairs by a back door. When we went there for therapy, I could leave ours home for Sam. (Incidentally, it would be a worthwhile public relations strategy for supermarkets to adopt this practice as well and provide a few wheelchairs for customers who need them.) The fact that we didn't have to cart the chair to the hospital not only helped my back, but it also aided Const in that she could feel some measure of independence by leaving it behind. We both were glad when she started to get around with a cane and leg brace for short distances.

I say this in spite of a couple of unexpected consequences this new achievement had for me.

Const liked to use the cane for purposes it was not intended. I've noted how she would scrape up clumps of dog hair with it and push them into tidy little piles for me to clean up. If left to my own devices, I would never have known that the offending stuff existed. I was sure it couldn't be seen with the naked eye, and was at a loss figure out how Const had noticed it. Then I figured it out. She hadn't really seen it; she just knew from experience that it would be there.

She also tried to hook Sam out of her wheelchair with her cane (to no avail), but her favorite pastime was whacking me on the calves with it. The rollicking grin on her face as she did so was worth the few times I felt any discomfort.

The biggest drawback to the cane was that it would often manage to disengage itself from Const and strategically place itself where I would stumble over it or kick it unknowingly. Then there were the times I had to spend an hour trying to find out where she left it.

Const hated the leg brace with a passion, but it did more good than harm. It kept her knee from locking when she walked, although her ankle was kept in one position and got precious little exercise. We tried special knee braces and elastic bandages rather than that big heavy monster that fit down into her shoe, but the molded brace worked the best, at least while she was still weaning herself from the wheelchair.

We both looked forward to a day when the brace might not be necessary, but there was a long way to go.

Seven

The Metal Spatula, and Other Household Discoveries

Lord Almighty, I thought, *what am I doing?* I was cleaning the bathroom sink after washing my hands, just as Const had demanded. I was becoming domesticated!

I told myself that this housework stuff had to stop. But I knew it wouldn't, since it had to be done and I was the only one capable of doing it.

As a professional consultant, I pretty much call my own shots in the workplace. And while I'm fortunate that my job permits me to remain at home most of the time, being indoctrinated into the Constance Collins school of housekeeping was not on my agenda.

I like to think that I sometimes find myself doing things Const's way because in certain cases, her procedures are the best ones. An example was when it finally struck me that it's not a good idea to hang dish towels in a clump on the rack, since they don't dry that way. Const had not said anything, but had spent an inordinate amount of time properly displaying them in the hope I would eventually get the message. I did, and began following her lead. However, I also like to think that I've come up with a few ideas and innovations of my own.

For instance, I'll bet the average housewife doesn't know how handy the metal-bladed spatula is. The rubber-bladed one does a nice job of cleaning out sticky bowls, but that's about all it's good for. "Oh, yeah?" some woman is probably scoffing, "what about frosting a cake?" Well, I don't eat enough cake to have a rubber-bladed spatula cluttering up the kitchen drawers.

The metal one is a handy tool for everything short of ladling out soup. I fry bacon, stir potatoes, soup or canned beans with it, and then use it to clean the burned stuff off the bottom of pots. It's one of the most valuable kitchen tools, and it minimizes the dishwashing. This in itself was an important discovery for me, since doing the dishes was one of my least favorite chores.

While I was cooking, I learned to run some hot water in the sink and wash or soak bowls, pans, pots, dishes and utensils as soon as I was finished with them. (If you have a dishwasher, I can't help you— we threw ours out long ago when we realized that several sets of dishes would roost in there.)

One of my other little triumphs came when I

solved the sugar bowl problem. Like many sugar bowls, ours had a bottom on it one third smaller than the top. It was easy to tip it over on the shelf, and I could swear it had legs and deliberately moved to a spot where it could be bumped. Over it would go, and I would spend five minutes cleaning up the gritty mess, only to have it tip over again once I had finished.

I solved the problem by doing what I considered to be a pretty clever thing—I dumped the sugar back into the sugar cannister, washed the bowl and returned it to the shelf empty. We never used much sugar anyway. Only the ants would be unhappy, if they ever showed up.

Const didn't seem to appreciate this as a major victory, however. Her comment was, "Why didn't you just move the sugar bowl down one shelf among the salt and pepper shakers?" That was okay, though; my little flashes of inspiration were their own reward.

I learned the hard way to cover beans when heating them in the microwave oven—they tend to erupt upon the slightest provocation. Don't heat uncovered German potato salad in the machine either, unless you're looking forward to spending the afternoon cleaning up.

The microwave is a great tool for heating things, provided you don't try to heat them in a metal pan. I don't know the principle behind microwave cooking, but I do hate plastics in most forms, and I don't like having to heat food in plastic containers. The best alternative I could come up with was to simply put the food into a regular clay or ceramic dish. The dish would be hot coming out of the oven, but it kept the food hot longer while I finished preparing the rest of the meal.

Getting fuzz off of blouses and other clothes is a task I could never figure out to my satisfaction. Socks are a big culprit, and although I found it would help when I turned them inside out before tossing them in the wash, this did not solve the problem. The best I could come up with was to use my electric razor for the job. This was the same razor I had once forbidden Const to use to clean the fuzz off of clothes.

I guess having to pull the blades out and clean them off is worth the effort. The only problem will be when she reads this and discovers what I did, and I have to apologize to her for not allowing her to use my razor in the same fashion.

Of course, some of the household strategies that Const did know about did not meet with the queen's approval. Laundry is a good example. Every time I brought a load up, Const would manage to fish something white out of the clothes basket and examine it.

"Are you using two cups of bleach?" she inquired upon her first laundry inspection.

"Just one," I responded. Frugality is one of my most cherished virtues.

"Look at the collar on this shirt." She held it up with her good hand for me to inspect.

I had to admit the shirt looked a little grey, but bleach wears out clothes faster than taking them down to the river and pounding them on rocks. At least this was my experience when I had to do my own washing in the navy. Of course, in the navy I hadn't had an inspecting officer like Const.

I realized I couldn't hide it from her, and since I didn't have any other solution, I began to toss in one and three-quarters cups of bleach. She quit holding the clothes up to her face to examine them...case closed.

Then there were the tasks where my own ingenuity and skills were woefully inadequate to tackle a problem. In one case, however, this actually led to a big leap forward for Const.

One day she announced that she wanted me to help her negotiate the steps down to the basement. I was pleased, but surprised; I knew her well enough to realize that something had to be motivating her to let me help her go down there.

At the time, Const was getting along very well with just a cane for support. While she favored her left leg, she was walking around the house instead of using the wheelchair. She had also practiced on steps for many hours during her outpatient therapy at the hospital, and the therapist had announced that she could test the basement steps at home when she felt equal to the task. Until now, she hadn't felt ready.

I decided to stay behind her while she went down the steps and control her efforts with a safety belt, a heavy, woven cotton apparatus which encircles the waist and allows the caregiver a formidable grip. Once the other person attains a level of confidence, the caregiver merely keeps his fingers under the belt and allows the patient freedom to do her thing. A stroke victim must be allowed as much latitude as possible to help herself, and Const was no exception.

(Of course, neither of us had any thought of abandoning the safety belt until absolute confidence was attained, not only by Const, but by myself as well.)

Halfway down the steps, while Const held onto the handrail, I was starting to have grave misgivings about having undertaken this adventure. If she misstepped, I doubted if I could hold back her momentum and weight and keep myself from catapulting after her.

Temporarily calling a halt to our progress, I eased myself around her and tried guiding her from below. This, I quickly determined, was worse than being above and behind her. I had even less control, and the end of the railing was only one step away, so we'd have nothing for support for the last three steps.

"Honey," (she always calls me this whenever she knows I'm struggling with something) "the therapist was always beside me on the steps."

There's only room for one and a half people on the average set of basement steps, but I compromised. I kept one foot on the step below and one on the same step she was on. My fancy footwork and her laughter at my awkward positioning kept us going, and we finished the initial journey.

The laundry room was a disaster area, and I briefly entertained the notion of steering her away from it. Deep in my heart, though, I knew better. Once she was down there, I knew we were going to have a white glove inspection.

She grabbed her cane and made for the laundry room. She poked at a towel laying in a corner and fished one of my shirts off the clothesline. Then she checked the controls on the clothes washer. "Your last load was whites." She pointed to the dial setting, which was on "cold." "You wash whites in hot water."

This was news to me. The doggone box of soap said you could wash all clothes with it in cold water. When I explained, she said she had a bridge I could buy in Brooklyn, too.

She continued her rounds, and nothing escaped her attention. Within minutes she had two weeks of steady work lined up for me. But as it turned out, this was not the reason she'd decided to come down the stairs.

To cheer her up, our daughter gave Const a pretty blouse. The size that appeared on the label was right, but either the cutter, seamstress or designer had run amok, and it fit like Omar's tent.

Our son-in-law's mother took it home and sewed an inch off the sleeves and sides, but it was still much too large. As Const set out for the sewing machine, I realized her true motive for getting down to the basement.

My only success with sewing consisted of having attached a button to a shirt. I used one of those little gizmos that slip through the eye of the needle and guide the thread (I pulled the device through the eye and presto, the needle was threaded). Then I held the button in place until I got two strands of thread through the shirt to hold it in position, and kept pushing the needle through until I was satisfied the button was securely fastened. Luckily, no one pulled my shirt open to see what kind of a mess I'd made — other than Const.

My one attempt at darning a sock was an unqualified disaster; I couldn't get anything more than my toes into it after I'd finished. I quickly decided it was smarter for me to buy new socks than to try to repair old ones, and until Const led me to the sewing machine that day I had given it a wide berth.

"Find something to sit on," she told me as she draped the blouse over the table near the sewing machine and settled onto the bench.

Fortunately for me, the speed control and bobbin upper-downer were on the right side of the machine, where her right hand and foot could control them. Without the full use of her left hand, however, she could not operate the machine and guide the material too. If you can visualize two people sitting at a sewing machine with one doing nothing but guiding the material while the other one operates the machine, you have a good idea how we got the job done.

When we had finished, Const was pleased with the results, and the blouse fit her pretty well. I was pleased that she was pleased. Mostly, though, I was pleased that I had come away without any stitches in my fingers.

Going back up the stairs was easier than coming down. I was put in command of the cane and stayed behind her, bracing her for support. This went so well that after a few more trials, she decided to try it without my assistance. This was a big milestone in her recovery effort, but a difficult one for me. I had to stay a couple of steps in front of her and be prepared for anything. The therapists really had done their job well, but I could not afford to relax.

Still, this progress was cause for a major celebration. And to think that if I had known how to sew, Const might never have been motivated to tackle those basement stairs.

Of course, there were those household problems without any apparent solution. I'll mention one of them, and would welcome any suggestions from anyone who has found an answer.

The fiends who invented the vacuum cleaner should have designed a better way to empty it. While I struggled to vacuum the carpet to no effect, the wheelchair commando would zip past me and say, "Empty the bag, honey."

Emptying a bag from a vacuum cleaner is like spitting upwind. Wait until afterwards to take a shower—a film of dust settles over your entire body as you struggle to detach it from the unit. Once it is out, you can't control the dust, hair, rug fragments, and whatever else is in there. Don't empty the bag outside if there is the slightest breeze, and don't empty it inside unless you plan to dust the entire house. Disposable vacuum cleaners seem to be a good idea to me.

Being a caregiver is not easy. It involves learning and practicing the skills of a nurse, a housekeeper, an accountant, and a handyman while still maintaining all the old responsibilities.

In order to be most supportive of and helpful to the stroke survivor, the caregiver must first consider the stroke survivor's personal strengths and limitations, and what that person must do in order to take care of him or herself. Caregiving can go on for a long period of time, and it is not wise to start out by trying to be a superman.

Help and support are available for caregivers. All a person has to do is ask for it, and learn what kinds of resources are available. This is no time to act like a martyr—that will only lead to bitterness and resentment later. The caregiver needs to set aside some personal time each day. Hobbies, fun activities and friends should still have a place in the caregiver's lifestyle. It is essential that the caregiver take care of his or her own physical and mental health. As a sense of humor is helpful for a stroke survivor, it is equally beneficial to a caregiver.

The stroke survivor and the caregiver need to be open and honest with each other in expressing thoughts, frustrations, and feelings. Together they can set reasonable goals for the future and recall cherished memories from the past. They must function as a team and work to help each other maintain a sense of hope.

Eight

The Return of Luigi

It was not until five months after Const's aneurysm surgery, and three months after her stroke, that I was ever more than ten feet away from her. Then I began to sense that we both needed some time to ourselves, so I went out and played nine holes of golf. It did us both some good.

Our marriage has always been strengthened when we have been faced with adversity; it has been when things were going smoothly that we have had some friction. I suppose we've had the normal number of tranquil and fractious spots—it only seems like we've had more than anyone else sometimes. In the last few months our problems seemed to be diminishing as Const continued to recover, so it was time for both of us to recharge our batteries somewhat.

By this time, Const was maneuvering with the cane some of the time, and other times without it. The wheeled beast was still a part of our lives; Const used it when she tired and when dressing and undressing. She also needed it when she wanted to haul items from one destination to another. I was trying to wean her away from the wheelchair completely, but it was too soon for such a measure.

Her wrist was weak, but it was starting to respond. The swelling in her hand, which she experienced every morning, was coming under control with the use of hot and cold baths, a wrist support brace, and the use of an isotopic glove.

The glove was an ugly black and appeared to be made of a stretchable synthetic material. A therapist had tested it out with Const, explaining that it would be uncomfortable and not too sexy, and when she agreed to use it, permission was received from the doctor. It helped, but did not really solve the problem of the swelling.

The use and appearance of her hand was very important to Const, even though she tried not to let on to me. But when she thought I wasn't looking, I saw her studying it.

There were two things Const wanted most out of life. One was to be able to walk normally, and the other was to be able to use her hand. At one point, when she was feeling somewhat discouraged, she told me she would settle for just being able to walk. I replied that I didn't want to settle for that; 100% recovery was what we had to shoot for. She nodded in agreement, and the hard work she'd put in since then was paying off.

Only three months after the stroke she was very

close to regaining control of her fingers and thumb. The thumb wanted to close ahead of the fingers, but I knew that if we talked to it some more it would respond, and that the weakness of the muscles in her hand would eventually disappear.

At this point she could pick up a very light object, weighing an ounce or less, and carry it twenty feet before dropping it. It had made our week when she was able to reach that goal. Then one day her left hand helped her right do a small chore without any special effort on her part. She didn't have to talk to it or force it, it just did it without any coaxing. Achievements like these were very encouraging to both of us. It was only a matter of time before she renewed her acquaintance with Luigi.

Const is a Nintendo videogame freak, and she and Luigi (a character in a game called "The Mario Brothers") were pretty close until she had suffered her "accident." Const had no problem beating me, even when I had Mario, the competing character in the game, working overtime. After her stroke, however, her video ability was gone.

When she first decided to try Luigi again, her left thumb, which was necessary for her to use in order to play the game, just couldn't handle it. A week later she was able to maneuver him around a little, but ran out of time before she could complete the first segment of the game, or "world." She continued to persist, however, and soon she could travel through an entire world and go on to the next one. I began to look forward to the day when she would be back to beating me.

I encouraged her videogame addiction. She has always been a fierce competitor, and maneuvering Luigi was excellent exercise for not only her thumb, but her whole hand. I tried to set goals for her, even though it's not my nature to be a taskmaster. Still, I did it for the great reward of seeing Const's progress.

Her spirits and determination were mostly very high, and for the most part she had come to grips with the fact that it would take time to recover her abilities. We were both told this explicitly right after the stroke, but in the beginning she apparently blocked it from her mind.

As has been mentioned, the general view is a patient will recover most control in the first six months after a stroke, and then continue to improve for the next two years. After that, there might still be some small breakthroughs. I knew that if it was at all possible, Const would succeed in a total recovery. I may have had to encourage her at times, push her a little at others, but I never knowingly gave her false hope. She had to have the drive inside of her, and my role was to spur it on.

I recognized my position early on after her stroke: I was the one person who had to make himself available twenty-four hours a day while she recuperated. That kind of closeness can test a relationship, but if I said or did things that upset her, I was only trying to help. At times it took little to provoke her, but that began to pass after awhile, and in fairness to her, I have to admit that I was at least as difficult to live with as she was.

Shortly after an individual has suffered a stroke, the stroke survivor and family begin to comprehend the change and loss it has caused in their lives. It is very normal and natural for all of those who were affected by the stroke to go through a process of grieving.

The grief process is a healthy and even desirable thing. If a person doesn't go through it, the pain of the loss may remain and be unresolved until that person is allowed (or allows him or herself) to grieve properly.

This process is similar to what a person goes through when they experience any other great loss in life, including death or divorce. There is no prescribed amount of time needed for a person to go through the grieving process, or an exact order that a person follows through the stages of grief.

*The five stages of grief, as defined by Elizabeth Kubler-Ross in her book, **On Death and Dying**, are denial, anger, bargaining, depression, and acceptance. These stages are often experienced by stroke survivors and their families.*

Denial is a temporary state of shock. It is during this stage that the person needs to collect him or herself and allow reality to settle in.

Anger comes on when the individual feels rage and resentment over what has happened. Anger could be self-directed, or directed towards others. This may be a difficult stage for families to accept or tolerate, and short visits may be helpful to avoid becoming a part or the focus of the anger process. At the same time, it is important to keep in mind that this stage is the time when the person may be in most need of support.

Bargaining is the stage where a person seeks to escape what has happened. A person may make promises to God or a higher power, hoping to change the unchangeable.

Depression is a stage where the person can no longer deny his or her condition. The stroke survivor may have feelings of uselessness, and starts to sense his or her loss.

Acceptance occurs when the person comes to grips with the reality of the situation and begins to develop a sense of peace and the ability to get on with life.

Hope is present through all of these stages.

Although depression is a very normal part of the grieving process, if a person becomes absorbed in this state and allows it to drag on and on, it can contribute to further impairment, both physically and emotionally. An individual who is clinically depressed will frequently express feelings of helplessness, hopelessness, and despair. The stroke survivor may appear very fatigued, and be uninterested in the activities of daily living. The person may also seek isolation from others, demonstrate very low self esteem, and be very self-critical.

When a person is stuck in the stage of depression, professional help is advisable. Since so much of stroke rehabilitation involves being active in therapy and working very hard to regain physical strength, depression will hinder this process and affect the overall recovery of the individual.

Counseling or psychotherapy can help the person through the period of depression. The counselor can assist the individual in working through areas of grief.

When depressed, a person tends to have a very negatively distorted perception of him or herself, others, and the rest of the world. Psychotherapy can help the person to challenge these negative distortions about life and encourage a reframing of the situation in a more realistic and positive way. The individual can be given tools which will help him or her challenge a negative thinking process. If psychotherapy by itself does not help the person, antidepressant medication may be prescribed by the individual's physician.

By conquering the challenge of depression, the stroke survivor is able to get on with the recovery process and develop a more positive outlook for the future. When the caregiver or family member works through depression, he or she is also able to become more functional and positive towards life. Both the stroke survivor and the caregiver will need to work together to find out what their new purpose or direction in life will be.

When a person is faced with the challenges that Const was, emotions can run high, and a normal sense of independence and privacy can be greatly disturbed. One of the most difficult times was whenever I had to help her in and out of the tub or shower. If she was going to break down, it was just before her bath. My heart went out to her, but there was nothing I could do to make things different. If I stayed away while she got in and out of the shower and she slipped and fell, things would have been much worse for both of us. Unfortunately, her modesty had to be sacrificed somewhat for her general welfare.

Unprepared!

I'm not a smooth talker; I doubt if I could sell stoves to the Eskimos. I like to attribute my lack of eloquence to being too honest. More likely, I just don't think fast enough on my feet. It wasn't long before I had all kinds of "shoulda saids" and "shoulda dones" tucked away in my head for future use.

The best way I found to encourage her was to keep notes, mental and written, of her progress, and to point out in vivid terms just how far she had come in the past week or two. For instance, I reminded her that opening a door with her left hand might not seem like much after she had mastered the task, but it was something which had been beyond her capabilities not too long ago.

We were lucky in that Const never lost the ability to speak. In observing other patients at the various treatment centers, it seemed to me that those hardest hit were the ones who had lost their ability to communicate verbally. Those who care for these stroke victims face an even greater challenge than I did, and I developed the greatest admiration for them and their ingenuity in helping to initiate forms of silent communication. For even though Const was just as articulate as before the stroke, I found I needed to invent some signals in addition to our "love code" to help her keep her sense of pride and well being.

Since the left side of her face had lost much of its sensitivity, a piece of food could lodge on that side of her mouth when she ate and she would never know it. The first time it happened, I instinctively wiped it away for her, but it became apparent that this served to remind her of her condition and demoralize her.

After I realized why she had become upset, I asked her to look at me once in a while during meals. When our eyes met I would surreptitiously wipe the corner of my mouth if she had a bit of food showing. It worked wonders for her, and the problem was solved.

Of course, I was not the only one who had been guilty of an occasional lapse of tact. While the therapists were tremendous, they sometimes said things that Const did not take well. For instance, one told her she was young to have a stroke. This upset her, and my belief that divine providence is impossible to predict was confirmed when, during grocery shopping, we met up with a young lady who had been born with a stroke. Const had engaged the girl in conversation when she noticed the molded cast on her leg, much like the one she herself wore. Const hid hers under slacks, but this girl had hers in full view. I tried to convince Const that it was all a matter of conditioning, but she still remained reticent to go out in public with her wheelchair, cane, or leg brace.

Many people were eager to help with doors when they saw a Laurel and Hardy act like ours going on at an entrance. It would probably help any victim confined to a wheelchair for the first time to be advised that strangers will react in one of four ways: they'll sneak a peek, look away, pretend not to notice, or rush up and see if they can help.

It was a constant job of mine to persuade my wife to get out more. What I had on my side was the fact that she had always been too much of an extrovert to get into a rut and turn into a recluse. And once she did get out, even to go grocery shopping, she would start to be her old self. The hard floors which increased her chair speed always brought a smile flickering over her face. Before I knew it she would be whizzing down the aisles, and if something was too heavy, or she couldn't reach it, the cane would start waggling in the air and I'd have to hurry and catch up or she would come racing back and smack me one on the calf with the cane, laughing heartily.

When I started going out with Const after her stroke, I noticed how most people look away from those in wheelchairs, and are often embarrassed by the incapacities of a handicapped person. Const set out to make up for all of them. If a person in another wheelchair did not mind some social interaction, she would wheel up and compare stories. At first I was concerned this might be callous, but I saw that the conversation between her and the other person would become quite animated. The therapeutic value for both parties was something to behold.

Perhaps the toughest thing for her was to meet old friends who had known her before her "accident." They remembered her as someone full of life and energy, bubbling with enthusiasm, and while she still had these qualities, it took some time before friends became comfortable in her company once again. Her natural charm would soon put them at ease, though, and after her initial anxiety she would end up having an enjoyable visit.

The outing I worried about most was when Const agreed to accompany me to the little shop where the first symptoms of her stroke had become obvious. "Are you absolutely certain you want to go out there?"

I asked her, concerned about how well she would handle such a strong reminder of the thing which had so radically changed her life.

She nodded, but I was not at all convinced she wanted to go through with it. However, I did know her well enough to realize that while she might be afraid, she would face this potentially traumatic event just to satisfy herself that nothing would happen to her again. We spent a good half hour there, and the feelings she must have had were not discussed between us. I suppose she feels there are some things best left unsaid, and I know there are times when silent support is the best thing I can offer her.

Nine
Goodbye Wheelchair!

Whenever a traumatic event like a stroke takes place, the victim, and to some degree the caregiver, can go into a form of shock. This condition can last for quite some time, as long as six months in some cases. And when the shock finally wears off, a state of depression can follow.

Const, four months after her stroke, only then began to fully realize what she had been through and what she would face in the future. The degree I had been in shock had not been as great, and consequently had worn off much sooner. Shock, as I see it, is nature's way of protecting you until you are able to cope.

The most noticeable sign of Const's emergence from this state of shock was her inability to speak about tender subjects without tears and a quavering voice. Fortunately, she never lost control of her emotions, and her sense of humor remained intact. There were some periods of depression, but they were normal considering what she had had to face.

The medication her doctor had prescribed to ease pain and allow Const to relax and sleep better was a great help. She had begun taking it when she started going to therapy.

Her pain was stroke related. Tendons in the shoulder ride in grooves, but due to the flaccid nature of Const's muscles since the stroke, her tendons could slip out of place and cause pain. Before she would take the medicine, however, the doctor had to assure her it was not habit forming; my wife is strong willed enough that she would rather have lived with the pain than taken that risk.

Including this painkiller, Const had to take three kinds of pills a day. It soon became a problem to determine whether she had taken her pills. I placed the bottles high in the cupboard, out of reach of our inquiring little grandchildren, and each morning I set out the required daily dosage on top of the bottle caps. The plan worked very well, except that there were times when I forgot to make sure she'd taken her medication and had to get out of bed to check to see if the tops of the caps were bare. Sometimes they weren't.

As I'm sure you understand by now, being a caregiver entails many different jobs and roles. I didn't mind the responsibility of keeping track of her medications, or even most of the household chores, but when she started feeling well enough to have visitors, I came to dread the proclamation "Company's coming," because I knew what that meant for me.

My housekeeping skills were not that bad, but were still far from professional. Const could perform chores with half the time and effort I could, but she tired out quickly because of her loss of muscle tone. The words "company's coming" would be followed by her wheelchair roaring out of nowhere, her cane waggling to direct me toward areas of the house that needed cleaning. I might have scrubbed the bathroom floor the day before, but it would have to be done all over again. Either that or I would suffer the wrath of an irate woman.

"And this time, get behind the toilet, wipe down the edge of the tub, and empty the wastepaper basket." You'd think people were coming to inspect the bathroom, not to visit with her. So I'd spend the better part of a day housecleaning in anticipation of the visit, and the first thing out of her mouth when they arrived would be "Please excuse the way the house looks." Const, myself, and our guests were all aware that the house was probably cleaner than the one they just left.

But there was another part of preparing for company that I disliked even more than the housework. The following sentence was one I dreaded hearing:

"Help me put these earrings on."

"Okay," I'd answer as enthusiastically as I could. Putting on earrings is not a two person job. Try pushing those little needle-like things through a microscopic hole in someone else's ear yourself and you'll see what I mean.

Whenever I was forced to perform this duty I

would remember that I had my two granddaughters to thank for it. Kathi had prodded Const to get her ears pierced just like hers were, and Karen soon took up the cry. Grandma tried to feign fear of being hurt, but the girls assured her there was nothing to worry about.

"What do you think, Grandpa?" Const asked me.

"If that barbaric ritual will please you and the girls, who am I to stand in the way of your satanic pleasure?" Actually, this was my way of saying I didn't care. At the time it seemed like a harmless bit of female vanity, but I would come to regret not taking a stronger position against it.

It is almost impossible to handle one of those little baubles, much less manage to aim it at the ear, hit the hole, and keep it aimed straight until it comes out the other side. Putting the one in Const's right ear required standing as close as possible in front of her; the left ear worked best if I was behind her. How far I had come...I was struggling to help put on earrings when my concern used to be getting rid of the things so I could nibble on a girl's ears.

While in the process of struggling with the tiny bits of jewelry I once wondered aloud about what had happened to Const's clip-on types, or the ones that screwed on like little "C" clamps. She told me she had thrown them all away, claiming that they hurt her ears. Well, the little tiny kind hurt *my* pride.

But when I thought about it, I was happy she was concerned about her appearance. It was an indication she was not giving up on herself.

In fact, she was making new strides all the time, even to the point where she was able to help out on some of the household chores. She began to insist on helping with the dishes, making the bed, vacuuming and dusting. This gave me time to do one of the things I do best...nothing.

Recovering from stroke is a task that encompasses the entire life of a stroke survivor. In order to foster the positive attitude that is so vital to progress, it is important to allow the stroke survivor to be as independent as possible, to make choices and exercise control over his or her life. The individual should also be encouraged to maintain his or her normal role within the family unit.

The roles of parent, spouse or friend don't change because of the stroke, and need to be maintained throughout the recovery process. This may be difficult for the caregiver, however, since that person may develop a sense of role reversal. For example, where a daughter may be used to being cared for by her mother, she may find that she has come to feel like a mother to her own parent. As in the Collins' case, a husband may have to learn domestic duties that have been carried on in the past by his wife. No matter how the responsibilites change, however, the family role of the stroke survivor must be preserved.

When I was doing housekeeping tasks alone, washing dishes was my priority. The rest of the chores could wait. This was my thinking on the subject: Knowing the bed will get messed up again as soon as you climb in, why bother making it? And although vacuuming is supposed to reduce wear and tear on the carpets, I submit that the goal of the carpet industry is to have you wear them out with constant cleaning so they can sell you new ones. As far as dusting went, our grandchildren enjoyed playing tic-tac-toe and were learning sportsmanship all over the furniture.

Const didn't see things my way, and once she felt strong enough, she was welcome to whatever chores she could manage. In all seriousness, though, I reminded myself to resist the temptation to fall back into lazy complacency when it came to housework. My experiences had made me fully appreciate the scope of demands that most women deal with. Consider that the roles of mother, housekeeper, cook, wife, and income provider are all pretty much full time jobs, and you'll wonder too how they manage to cope.

After years of watching my mother and then my wife perform endless chores, it still never occurred to me they might appreciate a little help, and it took Const's stroke to open my eyes. Perhaps this was partly their fault; they rarely let it be known that they needed any help.

While Const was struggling to be helpful, I did not push her. She was desperate to make herself as useful as possible, so I constantly had to remind her to please ask me to help her with something rather than get angry and frustrated because her left hand wouldn't help her out.

One night we decided to make my favorite hotdish for dinner. (It is the only hotdish I will eat—most of the others I have been subjected to taste like heated dishrags soaked in kerosene.) I was busily peeling potatoes, and Const was trying to slice them. She eventually gave up, for which I was thankful; the spud was skidding around and I was afraid she might cut herself.

I heard her puttering around with a can of tomatos. Suddenly she let out a shriek, and I wheeled around to investigate.

"Look," she cried, "look, I can do it!" She began crying for sheer joy. She was able to hold the tomato can with her left hand and was opening it with a two-handed can opener! I tried to give her a hug, but she was already on the telephone to call our daughter Barb and give her the news. In this case, taking on a household task had proven to be wonderfully thera-peutic.

One of the biggest milestones was achieved a few weeks later, after she resumed doing these chores. Her last day of therapy finally arrived. She was apprehensive about it, and I could understand why; she had lost a great deal of her self-confidence right after her stroke, and had come to rely on the therapists and to enjoy the relationships she had formed over the past several months. Also, she knew that from this point on, progress would be up to the two of us.

I was confident she would continue on her road to recovery. In all the years I've known her, my Const had been able to do anything she'd made up her mind to accomplish.

She proved me right when, several weeks after therapy was over, she began to go without the leg brace. Not only had it felt very heavy to her, it had required her to wear special shoes which didn't suit her taste. I couldn't fault her opinion on how they looked, but the shoes did the job. She hated them, but she knew they had helped. Nevertheless, Const was eager to do without them.

Abandoning the brace allowed her to strengthen her ankle, which would help her to walk normally. She continued to improve, and finally we were able to return the wheelchair.

I wanted to get a bottle of champagne to celebrate, but our joy was tempered slightly by our unspoken feeling that we would sometimes miss the chair. At the time we brought it back, Const couldn't walk more than a couple hundred yards without tiring out. Still, the sense of accomplishment was worth the price. We had climbed another mountain. ("Price" might be a poor choice of words—our insurance company picked up the tab for the chair, and the initial billing showed she could have had it for another four months.) Soon my back was starting to feel like normal again, since I no longer had to hoist the contraption into and out of the station wagon.

Five months after her stroke, the swelling in Const's hand had gone down somewhat. She still wore the isotoner glove at times to keep it manageable, and the support brace for her wrist was only worn at night to protect her hand from damage while she slept.

Her sleep was still fitful, due to her inability to move easily. As a consequence, she would wake up after the least little struggle. She hated the shoulder harness she had to wear at night with a passion, but she put up with it in case it was doing some good.

Around this time Const got a new device from a

therapist called a neuromuscular stimulator. After a lengthy consultation with her doctor, she decided to give it a try. A battery pack hooked on her waist and delivered a shock impulse to sticky patches fixed on her shoulder. The purpose of the gadget is to pull the tendon back into the socket position through the use of electrical impulses. It really did move the tendon back to its correct location whenever it energized, but even after a month of day and night jolts, the string-like tendon kept returning to its out-of-groove position, so we gave up on the gadget. The unit was heavy, and we had to be sure it didn't accidentally get turned up too high, but Const was generally willing to try anything that might speed her recovery, and I did all I could to encourage this attitude.

Others noticed how I offered support to my wife during these difficult times, and I have to say that for me, perhaps the most difficult part of the recovery process was graciously accepting their sincere compliments. I like to believe that anyone placed in my position would have reacted in the same manner.

Const and I once touched briefly on this subject, and I know that if I had been the one who had suffered the stroke, she would have moved heaven and earth to help. I observed other spouses in our predicament, and while I had no idea how they handled problems at home, I saw that within the best of their abilities, every caregiver responded with all the love and expertise he or she had to offer.

That's really what marriage is all about, isn't it?

Ten
Call 911

Const had had her aneurysm problem in February, and she had been recovering steadily from the stroke that had knocked her down in April. Things were letting up nicely for us, and October and November were the two best months we'd had all year. We had settled into a routine, and Const's Christmas shopping was nearing its completion. (Notice I did not say "*our* Christmas shopping." This was one task over which I was glad to give her complete reign.)

We had no way of knowing that something was once again about to drastically disrupt our lives.

I am an extremely early riser by nature; four-thirty a.m. is time to get up for me. By five I was at my word processor, and would have until eight to accomplish something. After that, Const would be up, and I often wouldn't have another such block of private time for the rest of the day, so those early morning hours were somewhat precious to me.

As a result of my early schedule, however, I am usually ready for sack time by nine at night. Of course, I manage to sneak in an extra hour or so of napping now and then in a comfortable chair.

On November 26th I drifted off at about eight-thirty. At roughly a quarter to nine I heard Const calling me. A strange phenomenon had occurred recently; I used to be a sound sleeper, and took pride in my ability to sleep under any conditions, but after Const's stroke, I discovered that it took very little to wake me when she called.

I heard her softly cry out for me, and I came to. She was spread out on the floor in the front room.

"I fell," was all she said.

This was the one thing I had lived in fear of since Const's stroke. Using my training as a process engineer, I had spent a lot of time trying to eliminate any and all obstacles which could cause her to fall. The one factor I could not do anything about was Sam, who had an annoying habit of being underfoot, and I often worried he might cause Const to stumble. It turned out, however, that Sam was not the cause.

My first impulse was to help her up. Of course, picking up a one hundred and twenty-seven pound person from the floor is no small feat. I asked her if she remembered how the therapists had taught her to get up. (This was a fascinating aspect of her therapy to me; not once did any of the therapists suggest she might fall, they simply taught her how to get up.) She said she did, and tried to roll over on her stomach.

Her sudden shriek of pain brought Sam and Missy

running. I knew by her cry that she was seriously hurt. Either she had a broken bone or she had dislocated her hip.

We needed help. While a dislocation is painful, a break, depending on how and where it happens, can be much more dangerous, especially for someone who is on blood thinning medication. Fortunately, my ancient Navy first aid course had impressed upon me that by no means should I try to move an accident victim. The reasoning was that if a break had occurred, it could be sharp, and in trying to help, the bone could very well sever an artery.

"Call Barb," Const pleaded. But I knew our daughter was twenty miles away, raising three children, working several days a week in a hospital emergency room, and going to school for nursing.

"Not right now." I headed for the telephone and dialed 911. The operator answered immediately.

I told her my wife, a stroke victim, had fallen, and probably had a dislocated or broken hip. She took our address, and without me giving my name, asked me if I was Mr. Collins. Her computer had told her who I was.

"Don't move her, help is on the way. Are there any special problems we should know about? Are you alright?" I answered her questions, and she went on. "Turn on a porch or yard light," she advised.

This gave me something to do. I flipped on the yard light and porch light switches and then found the coachlight switches on the front of the garage. I peeked out as a squad car, lights flashing, drew up to the curb. It must have been no more than a few blocks away.

The policeman took out his notebook and started firing questions. He wanted to know our names, her age, how her fall had happened, our preference in hospitals, and whether I could prop the front door open. To his last question, I told him I would when the ambulance arrived—this was November in Minnesota, and I couldn't see keeping the doors open any longer than necessary.

Less than five minutes later, another squad car and an ambulance had pulled up. Four well trained men prepared to move Const. Almost immediately they produced a plastic board designed to immobilize an accident victim. They slipped it into place under her, and she was strapped down tightly from head to toe. Const did not let out a whimper, even though being restrained is something she cannot abide. Within minutes, the ambulance was off towards our designated hospital and I was being driven there by a neighbor.

My mind was a total blank; I was numb from everything that was happening. I wondered how she could have fallen in the middle of the room like she had. Remembering the cop's questions, I wondered if he had suspected me of pushing her. No, she had told him I was asleep at the time. My thoughts were less than completely coherent.

I had given our daughter Barb a quick call before leaving the house, and I couldn't have been at the hospital more than twenty minutes before she and her husband Bruce walked in. When I asked how they had found a baby-sitter so quickly at that time of night, she replied, "That's what neighbors are for," dismissing the topic in five words. Just like her mother.

Since Const was on a blood thinner, she could not be operated on immediately. After about a half hour, once x-rays had been taken and the results examined, a "Dr. Dave" told us her hip was badly broken. "We'll start her on vitamin K to thicken up her blood," he said, indicating this was a standard procedure. A patient can lose a great deal of blood during a hip operation.

He didn't have to tell me that between removing the blood thinner and the operation itself, Const was running the risk of another stroke. Any operation, as far as I understand it, brings with it some small risk of stroke, although no doctor is going to dwell on that when the patient has other things to worry about. Any tiny particle of debris that comes loose from the inner wall of an artery can cause it to happen. But it was a risk that had to be taken.

It was not until the following evening, after a blood test had been done, that the doctors felt Const's condition had stabilized enough to perform the operation. When she came out she was heavily sedated and put in intensive care. I did not realize it at the time, but her condition had been critical before, during, and shortly after the operation.

She had been through quite an ordeal; I counted twenty-two surgical staples in her leg when they were removed two weeks later.

The first days of recovery did not go well for us, and I was thankful when Connie, the therapist who had been such a help to Const right after her stroke, appeared with consoling information and support. Const was extremely susceptible to the drugs she was on after the operation; they put her in a world of her own. And while she was very mild and quiet when she was recovering from the aneurysm surgery, this time she was more disoriented, and sometimes became suspicious and even violent.

No matter where the telephone was hidden in the room, Const would find it and call me in the middle of the night. Once she called to discuss the wonderful dinner she'd just had with the governor, who happened to own the room she was in. You can imagine how I enjoyed being awakened at two in the morning to get this news, but this was not the worst of it.

Const called me one morning at five to inform me she never wanted to see me again. She was going to live with her sister who lives near Milwaukee, and I was never to visit. Something was very wrong.

I tried to placate her. "Honey," I began.

Don't you "honey" me," she scolded, "I mean what I said." *Bang*, down went the receiver. End of conversation. End of better than forty-three years. I was stunned, even with my memories of the previous experiences. She had spoken in a convincing and articulate manner.

I dialed the nurses' station right back. Unbeknownst to me, she had been reassigned to a room reserved for rowdy patients, which happened to be right by the nurses' station. I found out they had made the mistake of putting restraints on her, and she thought I had given my consent.

It took a good chunk of time and effort for me to

convince her otherwise. I talked fast, telling her I had nothing to do with her being tied up and explaining the hospital staff had done it for her own safety. When I finished, I thought the problem was over. Then I learned she had informed the doctor, whom she worshipped, that she would see him in court. It was several weeks before I could convince her the nurses use their own good judgment with patients who are in danger of hurting themselves. If there had been any way for her to have cornered the nurse who had restrained her, I'm not certain what would have happened. Despite her loving nature, she does not forgive such an indiscretion easily.

Then came the most difficult decision we would have to make during her recovery. Although she improving steadily from this latest trauma, she was once again immobile, and the hospital was ready to discharge her. There was no way I could handle her at home in her present condition. Maybe in several weeks, when she could help, but not now.

It was time to talk to the hospital social worker who had been assigned to us.

In some cases, a patient isn't ready to return home immediately after being hospitalized. There are other options, however, such as hospital-based acute rehabilitation programs, hospital-based care facilities, and nursing and convalescent facilities. The choice depends on three factors: what the physician and health care team recommends, the patient's potential for recovery, and what that individual's personal medical insurance company will cover.

Unprepared!

Those who have a good rehabilitation potential and can physically tolerate an aggressive rehab program are candidates for an acute rehab facility. In acute rehab, the person usually stays at a hospital facility for one to four weeks, depending on physical needs, and will be up and dressed every day. (Constance Collins went to an acute rehab facility after her stroke; the program referred to here is not intended for patients with hip fractures.)

In order to qualify for an acute rehab program, the individual must have a good prognosis for recovery and be able to tolerate three hours of therapy every day. Consider that even a healthy person would have to be in excellent physical condition to endure three hours of exercise, and you'll understand why acute rehab can be thought of as a kind of boot camp for stroke survivors. Comfortable clothes that are easy to move around in are recommended, along with comfortable athletic shoes.

For individuals who need a short term structured rehab program but can't tolerate three hours of therapy daily, an extended care facility may be the best option. This program is very similar to the one that the stroke survivor was on during his stay at the hospital, but therapy is done on more of an individualized pace.

When a person needs long term rehabilitation, has a poor prognosis for recovery, or has an insurance plan that won't pay for the other two options, a nursing care facility is often the alternative. Nursing homes have changed drastically over the years, and are no longer seen as "places where people go to die." Statistics show that a significantly greater number of people go there for a short period of time for rehabilitation and to regain strength prior to returning home rather than go to live out the final days of their lives. For medical purposes, and due to changes in the reimbursement system, shorter hospital stays have become the norm, and rehabilitation and recuperation is now often done in nursing facilities.

Each floor in the hospital has a social worker, and since we were on a different floor than when Const had been hospitalized for her stroke, our social worker was not Mary. It is the social worker's job to help things go smoothly for patients and their families. This woman readily agreed to find a nursing home to care for Const. However, the closest one with a bed available was twenty-five miles away. The social worker told us she had heard nothing but good things about it.

At this point, Const's frame of mind was fairly good. That she could handle the consequences of her injury without total emotional destruction was amazing to me. She was not yet in any condition for therapy.

Const agreed to a temporary stay at the nursing home provided I visited her every day, and an ambulance with two medics drove her out there while I followed in our car. The place seemed nice enough for the most part.

I kept my promise to come by daily, and after three weeks I took her home in time for Christmas, as I'd told her I would. By the nursing home's standards, she was not yet quite ready for home care, and I had to use up an entire tree filling out paperwork which assured the nursing home I wouldn't sue them if things did not work out.

Christmas was celebrated with all the trimmings, as I managed to handle the turkey, cranberry dressing, and all the rest. We sat at the dining room table with Barb and Bruce and grandkids Kathi, Karen, and Eric. Phone calls rolled in from Const's family and mine from across the country. I had to call a halt to it after awhile, since I could see Const was getting exhausted. Although she wanted to talk to everyone, the big bad ogre had to shut down communications for the day. A caregiver's responsibilities take on many forms, and the patient's good comes before any well meaning efforts on the part of others. I think they all understood, and they could always call again the next day.

It wasn't until several days after Christmas that I made an unexpected and disturbing discovery about the nursing home where Const had been. She had told me at some length about how horrible the place was for her, but it took some subtle prodding before she unloaded the whole truth on me.

I already knew the food was bad; they could screw up even something as simple as a baked potato. While their chicken soup was fair, the dumplings were chunks of cardboard biscuits soaked in broth. But I was aware of their substandard cuisine; I had taken several meals there.

The disquieting revelation, and I found it very, very difficult to come up with any acceptable reason for it, was that the nursing home expected Const to submit to showers and trips to the restroom helped by a male. And not even a male nurse, but a man whom I had reason to doubt had much of a background check prior to his hiring. It was the nursing home's practice to use minimum-wage workers of both sexes indiscriminately, apparently without thought as to the patient's modesty.

During all her health problems, I had been very careful not to subject my wife to embarrassment when I helped her into and out of the shower and on trips to the bathroom. Once I was satisfied she was in control, I left her until she called. A normal standard of decency requires a somewhat delicate protocol; that's simply common sense. Then I discovered that it was apparently normal procedure for strange males to assist her in a nursing home. This I could not accept.

You may say that nursing homes exist only to make a profit. Well, if that's the case, then the states should be monitoring them more stringently. It is far too late to help a person once his or her dignity has been violated; the trauma must not be allowed to happen in the first place.

Reflections of an Occupational Therapist, Part Two

by Constance S. Shaffer, O.T.R.

In this section, Constance Shaffer tells about her experience with Mrs. Collins after her hip injury.

I was on orthopedic rounds when I heard Constance's name mentioned and learned she had been admitted with a fractured hip after a fall at home. Total hip replacement was scheduled for the next day.

When my rounds were done I stopped by to say hello, but she was sound asleep. As I walked down the hall I ran into her daughter Barb, who was upset about the setback and nervous about her mother's upcoming surgery. I talked with her awhile, trying to reassure her. I said I would check back later when her mother was awake.

On my next visit I found Constance awake and in

the company of a number of family members. They were all nervous about the pending surgery, the possibility of a second stroke, and Constance's reaction to anaesthesia and medication. Her reaction to drugs had apparently been a problem when she had had surgery for an aortic aneurysm.

I tried to explain what to expect, and to alleviate some of their fears. I referred them to Constance's doctor for further information. "This isn't like having a stroke," I said. "She will have the operation to repair her hip, and then we'll get her up and going, probably the day after surgery. Physical therapy will start showing her how to walk again, but she already has good balance and can move her left foot, so it won't be like going back to where she was right after her stroke.

"Occupational therapy will probably see her on her second day. If she moves around without too much pain in physical therapy, they'll begin teaching her how to do her lower half dressing. The rehabilitation process won't be as extensive this time—she should be able to get back to her previous level of independence relatively soon.

"There will be some added complications, because she won't be able to bend forward or cross her legs until about three months after the hip replacement." I looked at Constance. "It'll take awhile to get back to where you were before your fall, but you'll get there if I know you." Constance was looking tired, so I ended my visit. I stopped in to check with her family periodically over the next couple of days.

I began seeing Constance for therapy on the

second day after her surgery. Unfortunately, her family's fears about the effect of the medications Constance had to take were somewhat realized; she was confused and disoriented. On that day she did not recognize me and was unable to concentrate or listen to instructions regarding the precautions she should take for her hip. We worked on using a reacher to help her put on pants, so that she could slip them over her feet without bending forward. Her confusion, the pain in her hip, and the leftover effects of her stroke were all working against her. Both El and Barb were there, however, and provided wonderful support for Constance.

This visit took place on a Friday, and by the time I came back to work on the following Monday things were going better. Her level of confusion had decreased and she was getting back to her old self. She still had problems remembering her hip precautions, constantly wanting to bend down or cross her legs like she did before the fall. I eventually was able to impress them upon her, however, with Barb's assistance. Constance began to show progress in being able to put on pants for herself using the reacher. I learned that walking was going slowly in physical therapy, as again Constance had extra obstacles to contend with because of her weak leg, which she had difficulty advancing, and her left hand, which prohibited her from being able to use a walker.

Because of her difficulty in getting around and the amount of assistance Constance required for self care, it was recommended that she go to an intermediate facility where she could receive continued therapies on a daily basis to get her back on her feet again.

It was agreed upon that Constance would be sent to a nursing home to recover. She still had all her motivation and desire for independence that she had after her stroke, so I knew this would be just a temporary stop and that she'd soon be home keeping an eye on El again.

A couple of months later I was walking through the halls when I looked up to see Constance and El coming towards me. She was just as bright and chatty as she had been before her fall. I've always felt that the most rewarding part about being a therapist is being able to see the patients, whom you saw immediately after a disabling incident, progress and regain control of their lives. Watching someone succeed in their fight to pick up an object, wave or shake hands gives the therapist an overwhelming feeling of self worth. Constance always made my day when she stopped in to say hello and gave me that wave.

Eleven

The Van

In the first month after Const returned home, there seemed to be a whole new set of difficulties facing us. This was the third time in a little over a year that she was trying to bounce back from a serious health problem, and I suppose we had both been worn down emotionally.

Connie's advice on how hip fracture victims could be subject to mood swings served me well, and helped me guard against losing my composure during some of the trying episodes that arose in daily living. I had to fight to contain anger at some of the problems that I thought could have been avoided.

Const has always been a more expressive person than myself. If I hurt myself, slip with a knife or accidentally smack my hand with a hammer, I tend to forget about it after the initial hurt fades, and I made the mistake of thinking that Const should adopt the same attitude in recovering from her hip injury. During those first days after her fall, however, her discomforts were expressed with long and frequent grunts and groans.

I didn't doubt for one minute she was hurting, but sometimes I wondered if it was necessary to announce it so much. If I was stupid enough to suggest she withhold some of her complaints, I got a lecture and was told to experience her problems and see how it felt. It didn't seem fair to me.

Looking back, I recognize how emotionally drained I was at the time. It had been about a year since Const's health problems began with her aneurysm. If that time was difficult for me, I can only imagine how hard it was on her. But I was, and am, no saint. I've learned that in the course of any long illness or period of recovery it is natural for a caregiver to have feelings of anger and even resentment.

Every caregiver has to find a way to vent these feelings, and generally I would recommend whatever works for that person. Keeping a punching bag out in the garage, taking time out to work on a favorite project, or (heaven forbid) doing housework are some of the ways a caregiver can let it all out in a healthy manner.

With any incapacitating affliction, mood swings can keep a caregiver dancing on a hot stove lid. In one instance, the person you're caring for may get upset because you stepped in and helped, and the next time he or she may flair up because you didn't volunteer. All I can advise is that you try to cheer up; it will get better with time.

As I mentioned earlier, I have tried to learn when to help Const and when to back off and let her struggle with a problem alone. We made a pact early on: I do not take over and help unless she asks. Still, I've had to make judgments based on my knowledge of Const and her mood at the time.

I never bargained for the challenges we faced, but there were no alternatives. After forty-three years of bliss, I was experiencing the other side of the marriage contract, the part that says "in sickness and in health." We had thought that the worst of our trials were over with Const's stroke, but her hip injury gave us a new set to overcome.

After the stroke, we had gotten a parking permit from the state which allowed us to park in handicap spots and to park for free at meters. (We never took advantage of this second benefit—our town does not have parking meters, and I wasn't about to drive to the city in an attempt to get back part of the five bucks we were charged to apply for the privilege.) There had been a tremendous amount of rigmarole to get the permit. First I had to write to the state to get information about it, then find a deputy registrar's office to get the forms, then fill them out and take them to a doctor's office for a signature, then wait for a flimsy plastic card.

When the card finally arrived, she noticed that it was good for eight months, and I was certain that she used its expiration date as a guide as to when she would be over the stroke. After her fall, however, we had to get a new one.

The new sticker was for a three year period. Const

saw the expiration date, and by the look on her face I could tell she was disturbed by it. She said nothing, but I knew this was a mental setback for her. All I could do was try to encourage her to prove the world wrong about her recovery time.

A more difficult thing to cope with was the return of the wheelchair. She hated it more than ever, but there was no choice in the matter; without it, journeys of any length would have been out of the question.

This second go-round with the wheelchair was made more difficult by a couple of added complications. Since her hip injury, Const was unable to get into our station wagon, the vehicle we had used to transport the chair after her stroke. The wagon was a four-door vehicle, and the doors were fairly narrow. Also, the fact that it was low to the ground made it impossible for her to enter.

At first, it seemed that our little red truck, my automotive pride and joy, was the solution to the problem. By draping a throw rug over the seat, Const was able to get into it by backing up as close as she could and then having me hurry around to the other side and tug on the rug until she was in the cab. There was also a handle over the door so she could use her good arm to help pull herself up. The strategy worked pretty well, but there was one remaining problem.

The first struggle with the wheelchair was during the spring and summer months, and now it was the middle of winter. When we went out, I had to load the wheelchair into the back of the pickup. Rain, cold and snow may not deter a mailman, but it was unfair for Const to have to sit in a wet or frozen chair.

I had to admire the fact that she never complained, even after we had gone sixty miles an hour down the freeway with the temperature hovering around twenty below, not including the wind chill factor. Not a word when I helped her into the chair, but after I had parked the truck and caught up with her in the warm building, I would find her busily scraping frost off its arms. The look on her face when she realized I was watching reminded me of a kid who had gotten caught with a hand in the cookie jar. She simply did not want to complain, but I couldn't have lived with myself if I'd allowed the situation to go on.

My first thought was that a van might be our salvation. As much as I resisted the thought of giving up my red pickup, I knew that I'd have to trade it in. However, if the truck had to go, then the station wagon would go along with it. We'd kept the car because Const had insisted, not wanting to travel in my truck. Now that the wagon was no longer practical, there was no reason to keep it—we needed two vehicles like Sam and Missy needed fleas.

I went to visit the car dealers and found that both the truck and station wagon did not offset the price of a new van. In fact, the inclusion of the wagon in the deal only made up for the lost value of the truck. Driving my red pickup off the showroom floor had destroyed a good chunk of its cash worth. I decided to try to come up with another plan, but I borrowed a van from the dealer over the weekend to test it out in case I couldn't find another way.

Then it came to me. If I put one of those covers on the back of the truck and kept the rear window open to heat the now enclosed bed, I'd have licked the problem of the frozen wheelchair. All I had to do was find out where to get the right kind of cover.

They came in two designs. The first kind laid flat over the sidewalls of the bed, and the other was built up to the roof of the cab, providing even more enclosed space. I had the larger one in mind. It would have kept the wheelchair, the walker Const had begun to use, and even Sam and Missy all out of the weather quite nicely.

One problem. Const had taken too great a liking to the van when I had brought it home for the weekend trial. She wanted it, and not a cover on the pickup. Now I knew why the dealer had been so cooperative in letting me borrow it.

I have a theory which may have nothing to do with being a caregiver, but which has a great deal to do with auto salesmen. When a husband and wife check out several showrooms in the search for a new vehicle, the salesman knows that the man is usually concerned with the functional and economy features, and that the woman is more often after looks. He also knows which one will generally prevail.

All I could do was try to hold off on a decision and see if she softened her stance, but I knew that I wouldn't be able to stall more than a week or so. I'd want to talk about planning some purchases from the new seed catalog for the spring planting of our garden, and wind up debating the van. A conversation concerning a call to the plumber would somehow become a van discussion. I knew it wouldn't let up until I declared a flat yes or no.

The Van

To put it succinctly, we became the proud owners of a van.

The trips back out to the automobile lots were as maddening as I expected. Unless you've just arrived from Moscow or Venus, you know the TV and newspaper come-ons for cars are just that. Somehow the salesmen are never informed about the great deals that are advertised as lurking all over the lots; they simply shrug when you ask about them. I expected this, but it didn't mean I wasn't still angered by it. But I knew what we needed, and found a suitable van. Then it was Const's turn.

She gave her conditional approval to my choice, conditional because she still had to reach an agreement with the dealer. My queen can drive a hard bargain, but she was up against a tough challenge. I have often thought the government should use car salesmen to train its diplomats—we'd send the Japanese trade officials home in their underwear. She got the best deal she could, and we brought the van home.

I eventually came to accept the beating we took on the trade-in, and even admit the new vehicle's good points. The wheelchair resided in it whenever we were at home and came out only during trips, and I no longer had to haul it out from the back of the pickup or struggle to get it out of the wagon. The van also had enough room for not only the chair, but the walker as well, with space enough left over for a bag of golf clubs. The ride was smoother than the pickup, so there were no more grumbles from Const when we hit a pothole, and its front wheel drive gave it good traction in bad weather.

143

Unprepared!

I often wonder what a large van is like to drive. Ours is what they call a "minivan." They've become very common, and I can understand why. Our minivan is a delight to drive, very practical and economical, and since you sit higher than you do in regular passenger cars, the field of vision is much better.

***

One saving grace which helped us tremendously through all of the dramatic changes in our lives was the aid and goodwill of family, friends, and many of the health care workers with whom we came into contact. While I was the major caregiver, I make no bones about it; all of these people were invaluable in our time of stress.

The doctors, of course, provided vital supervision, and when necessary they pulled the strings to make things happen. I've already talked about how Connie, Const's therapist, went above and beyond the call of duty, and there were other health care professionals who did so as well.

Our daughter Barb and her husband Bruce were very supportive, taking the twenty mile drive from their house to ours quite often. Dennis, our son, is four hundred miles away, and he would check in by phone. When Const was first stricken he came to be with us, and although his wife Maryanne wanted to accompany him, I was glad he realized that the last thing I needed at the time was another person to entertain.

Const has a twin brother named Manny, who is somewhat like her in temperament. He too has a tendency to chew on a subject until it is in shreds, and at first I thought it wise to caution him to always be positive around his sister, and not to dwell on any negative aspects of her situation. As it turned out, my worries were unfounded, and he was a great source of strength to her.

When Const was recovering from her stroke, Manny went out and purchased a headset for her that plays cassette tapes. He and Const share a great love of music, and although I am not a music lover myself, I have never stood in the way of their enjoyment.

The smiles flashing over Const's face as she listened were a joy to behold, and I knew they would not have been there if Manny hadn't given her this thoughtful gift.

While our relatives were wonderful, I was perhaps even more gratified by the gestures of friends and acquaintances, since they were often unexpected.

Right after Const's stroke I ran into Lou, a member of our church, in the hospital. Lou was a volunteer, and had last seen Const when she was being treated for her aneurysm. He was surprised to see me there, and I explained that Const had had a stroke.

Lou conveyed his sympathies. "My wife had one five years ago," he added.

"Gee, Lou, do you think you could tell Const that? No one would ever know your wife had a stroke!"

"I'll be up this afternoon," he assured me.

He did better than that. I only knew him as a nodding acquaintance, but he brought his wife along with him. Her appearance did a great deal to boost Const's morale at a very difficult time.

The first week we were home, Joe, a customer of my consulting business, brought over a huge pan of lasagna. It lasted several meals, and saved my meal planning sanity when I was struggling to adapt to taking care of Const. Joe and his wife rate a huge measure of appreciation.

I've mentioned that a neighbor drove me to the hospital after Const had fallen, but I neglected to say that he was a man I hardly knew. He had seen the lights of the ambulance and squad cars flashing outside and come to see if he could be of help. When the telephone rang, he stepped over to answer it. Barbara was calling back. He provided details of how Const had fallen and injured herself. I gathered he was being grilled as he shook his head at the phone. After a few moments he turned to me and said, "Your daughter wants to know which hospital." He relayed the information, then added, "She wants me to drive you over, and I'm not to take 'no' for an answer."

It has always been my nature to do for myself, and I felt capable of this simple chore. In fact, my first reaction was to feel insulted that my daughter hadn't thought me capable of driving. But then I realized that in the stress brought on by an emergency, it is better to back off and allow other people to do for you—it's impossible for you to determine just how fit you are to perform a given task. My situation was not too different from a drunken person insisting he was fit to drive. Looking back, I'm extremely grateful for the way my neighbor pitched in to help me during this time of crisis.

Of course, if a situation was not an emergency, I was always cautious about accepting help from others. If a friend or neighbor offered to do something for us, I would jot down their name and type of offer, but would be careful not to overuse the relationship. I had no doubt they were sincere in their willingness to help, though, and I was amazed and gratified how people responded when they perceived we were in need of their aid.

Twelve

Therapy in a Pail

The doctor had informed us that due to the stroke, Const's recovery from her hip fracture would take longer. Of course, the reverse was true as well; the rehabilitation for her hip injury would affect her stroke recovery. We'd been hit by lightning twice, the new pin and plate in her hip adding to the obstacles she had to work to overcome.

One of the results of her injury was the onset of shooting pains in her hip, which she referred to as "spasms." No amount of exercise or medication seemed to do any good, and she would pray for an uninterrupted night's sleep.

Concerned about the possibility of another stroke, she insisted the doctor answer her questions in an honest and straightforward manner. She did not like what she heard. Since she had already had a stroke, another one could happen. The blood thinning

149

medication that she was on would help prevent a new occurrence, but it in turn had its drawbacks. For instance, it could cause an ulcer, which if gone untreated could raise havoc because of the very fact it was thinning her blood. From Const's hip fracture, we were already all too aware of the increased risks which would result from any injury that might cause bleeding.

Even now we cannot say with certainty what caused her fall. Her doctor had said she had good bone density, and equated the impact to a force of about two tons. The resulting trauma must have blocked Const's memory of the events leading up to the fall, because she still can shed no light on what happened.

My inquisitive nature led me to form a hypothesis, however, and I now feel fairly certain that I have come up with the answer.

Shortly before Const's fall, we had installed new carpeting. Not shag, which is extremely treacherous for someone in my wife's condition, but still a deeper pile than the old stuff. I feel that this was a contributing factor.

Const also experienced problems walking because she was not able to put her left foot down heel first as people normally do. Her plastic brace which extended from her leg down into her shoe corrected this, but she was not wearing it at the time of her fall. Aside from being heavy and uncomfortable, we both had felt she could get along without it for short periods. Besides, there was the consideration that her ankle and foot would not strengthen while she used the brace.

Finally, Const has always been an energetic and vibrant person. She doesn't simply do things—she attacks them. It doesn't matter what she's doing; she puts all her energy and verve into a project, even if it's something as mundane as doing dishes. That was her strength in therapy, but perhaps this time her zeal betrayed her.

My conclusion is that without the brace, Const may have pushed herself a little too hard, caught her toe in the carpeting, and lost her balance. This theory is supported by the fact that she fell in a relatively wide open space in the front room; she always used the utmost caution around steps, doorways, furniture, and other obstacles. Her diligence was probably at a minimum on an open expanse of carpeting.

The most amazing thing to me through this new round of recovery, and one of the things I'm most thankful for, is that even Const's hip injury did not change her basic attitude. Naturally, there were some moments of despair, and some emotional outbursts. "Outbursts" may not be the best word for them, but when emotions overflow without warning, the caregiver has to deal with them in whatever way will douse the fire. I may be fortunate; in our house, these moments never lasted for much more than a few minutes. Reminding myself what Const was facing helped me get through them. It would throw even the toughest woman for a loop to consider that she might never walk normally again, might never again wear her favorite high-heeled shoes, never be without a cane or walker.

But after suffering an anuerysm, a stroke, and a broken hip within ten months, it was little wonder Const had a temporary loss of confidence, and she soon bounced back to the point where she eagerly took on new therapeutic challenges. In fact, she became quite eager to try new things to speed her progress—perhaps too much so.

After her fall, I walked a tightrope in deciding what I thought she could do and worrying about what she might try. In explaining this to Const, I told her that while I had confidence in her abilities, I wanted to share in her achievements. If I had to leave the house for a few minutes or longer, I didn't want to have to worry that she might hurt herself by doing too much. She accepted my reasoning, and understood that I wanted to have the opportunity to see what she was trying. Not that I am an expert; I just had to share in the experiment and be on hand in case it failed. Once she had mastered something new, I left her to it. Before long she was traversing the basement steps alone once again, without me walking backwards in front of her as a buffer.

I would urge her to accompany me when I had to go anywhere for an extended period of time, and it was worth the effort. I preferred to know where she was and how she was faring at all times. Also, I knew she would enjoy herself and be the life of the party once we reached our destination. If I had her personality and charisma I could become the President of the United States, or whatever else I chose. If you ever meet the queen, I'm sure you'll agree.

Const is a doer, not a dreamer, and she developed

many techniques in order to accomplish her ends. For instance, if a pot or kettle was too heavy to carry to the stove, she would never drag it over the cupboard, since that would leave marks on the surface, especially if the pot was aluminum. She had to find another way, so what she did was spread out a washcloth or dishtowel, put the pot on it, and then drag it to the stove.

She rigged up a device to hook onto her walker so she could carry things around with her. Following her lead, I found a plastic tray with straps in a hospital store that was intended for the job; Const could even haul a cup of java around in it. (She has always been a full-time coffee slurper.)

However, while she did her best to compensate for her disabilities with innovations like those I've mentioned, my wife never accepted that they would be permanent. Instead, she applied herself to every facet of regaining her former health. While doctors and therapists cautioned her that she would never regain all of her former physical abilities, she never let their pronouncements discourage her. As for my opinion, my money's on Const. Anyone who knows her and has seen her progress inevitably comes up with one word to describe her: "feisty." I've had the additional advantage of seeing how hard she works at her therapy, both at the hospital and at home.

One day Const was struggling to carry a salt shaker. I saw her hand was drooping, bent forward in a classic stroke victim's position. Instead of taking it from her, I had an idea which would help her towards her goal to do for herself.

I took her hand and straightened it into the proper carrying mode, then walked several feet with her, just holding her hand. When I turned it loose, the hand remained in position for a short time. She was encouraged by this, knowing the task was possible and that practice would build her endurance. If she saw even the slightest progress, she would redouble her efforts in therapy.

While I was down in the basement doing laundry, Const would exercise her hand and arm on the pulley system I built for her as she supervised me. It was always a big boost to see her progress, for both of us.

A two pulley system was needed for the type of therapy Const was doing, for a reason that may not be immediately obvious. The weight which is used for resistance (in her case, a bucket), must stay well clear of the operator so it won't bang into that person. The first pulley is located over the weight, and the other about four feet closer to the operator.

The pulleys themselves only need to be large enough to allow a chunk of clothesline to fit through them. Most basements have an open part of floor which is an appropriate place to put this contraption, and ours happened to be in the laundry room. The pulleys should be installed so they pivot to keep from tangling the rope, which is fed through them and tied to the weight on one end. A handle can be fashioned for the other end out of whatever is handy. (A piece of dowel or part of a broom handle will work just fine.) The handle should generally be about five inches long and not over one inch in diameter.

Even with an empty plastic bucket as the only

weight, Const had some tough sledding at first, but I kept encouraging her. I would add to the number of hoists Const would do each day (whatever I could get away with) and gradually slip more weight into the pail. At first I'd use an old clothespin, a bent nail, or the like. I knew Const was keeping an eye on how much was in the bucket, so by adding small items I figured she would begin to lose count so I could fatten up the pot faster. Before too long, she was adding stuff herself, and was pulling about five pounds worth of odds and ends.

Do you recall our love code? Three squeezes for "I love you?" Well, one night I got an impressive demonstration of how her work was paying off. With her left hand she gave me our sign, and I could not believe the strength it had. We were in bed, and it was dark, so I had to reach over and find her right hand just to make sure the left hand was the one which had squeezed mine. What a moment that was!

As her recovery proceeded at a fairly good rate, her sense of humor when we were alone also began to return. In front of others she was loaded with it, and it was not an act—that's just the way she is. But it was her increasing sense of humor when there was just the two of us that told me she was returning to her old self. Our old private jokes are expected, but the new and different comical jibes and observations finally began to return to her character.

For example, when she figured I needed some attention and headed for her cane to give me a love tap, I would keep moving it away from her in increments. Eventually she would threaten to throw something at me, but she took my teasing in good humor.

Once again, she was rebounding.

Thirteen
A Piece of My Mind

One day Vince, the man who bought the shop Const and I once owned, asked me if I found I loved my wife more since her health problems began. I struggled for an appropriate answer, never having put those feelings into words before.

We are one. What happens to her happens to me. We look forward to celebrating our forty-fifth wedding anniversary in August, and a lot more after that.

Ours has been a good life; we've had some wonderful moments, a lot of good ones and some not so good, and only a couple of very bad ones. Everything considered, I'm sure Const would agree with me when I say that I'd do it all over again.

I met Const when I was working at the Massey Harris Company, now called Massey Furgeson. Massey is a farm implement manufacturer which at the time was located in Racine, Wisconsin. As an Experimental

Engineer, I sometimes had to pass through the front office. This was something I looked forward to, since there were girls in the office.

One of them caught my eye, a friendly blue-eyed brunette. But whenever I saw her, she was with another blue-eyed brunette of about the same height and shape. Both were nice, but the first one seemed to laugh and smile a lot more than the other.

I had one major problem: I could only tell them apart when they were together. When I found one by herself, I was never completely certain which one she was.

A once in a lifetime opportunity arose when I saw them talking, then part company. Wasting no time, I hurriedly button-holed the right one and asked her out. She hesitated for the proper amount of time before agreeing. (I still love to tell people I had mistakenly picked the wrong one; Const has learned to take my teasing in stride.)

It turned out that my new sweetheart had just parted company with a fine fellow who always showed up at her home with a different automobile. It turned out that none of them belonged to him; he merely owned the lock pick.

Two years after our first date, on a beastly hot day in August, we were married. Const's sister was planning the same kind of caper, so it became a double wedding.

Since then, Const has given me two beautiful children, Dennis and Barbara, who grew up to be strong and well adjusted adults. They, in turn, gave us four grandchildren of whom we are very proud.

Const lives for these children, and they've been a big incentive for her to recover as quickly and thoroughly as she can.

In addition to working in an emergency room as a nursing aide, Barb is currently pursuing her nursing degree. She has the greatest enthusiasm for her work, and if I get her started she can fill the better part of a day regaling us with her adventures. No doubt her great interest in the health profession has contributed to her usual "A" results on her tests. With her husband, two school age children and one in nursery school, plus a dog and home to care for, her accomplishments are even more impressive. Her husband Bruce has been very supportive, and that has certainly been a big help. Both Const and I appreciate him; if he has a fault, it is workaholism.

In spite of my daughter's obvious love for her intended profession, I still can't imagine what drives a person to become a nurse. I suspect that prestige and financial considerations motivate some students studying to be doctors, though certainly not all. Nursing, however, is not a financially rewarding occupation, and the unconventional hours and swing shifts can disrupt a nurse's life. There has to be something more driving them, and while I see the excitement and pride Barb has in her work, I can't fully understand her enthusiasm. The enjoyment I derived from my career as an engineer came from the challenge of creating something, so I obviously am motivated by different things.

I say this in spite of how strongly I take an interest in helping restore Const back to health. All I can say is that it tore me up to see what happened to her, and I knew I had to do all I could to help her get back to being the vibrant, extroverted woman I had known. It seemed doubly unfair that she was struck down at a time when you're supposed to be able to relax and enjoy life. But with the help of the health professionals, some as dedicated as Barb, she has made great progress in getting back to where she was before, and I have had no trouble motivating myself to help her as much as possible.

A nurse, however, must administer to all who come under her care and treat every patient with compassion. By and large, the nursing aids and L.P.N.'s who have worked with Const have been able to show a considerable amount of understanding.

Perhaps one day I will ask a doctor or an L.P.N. if I can follow them around and learn the ropes; I'd like to be able to tell people more about their concerns.

The vast responsibilities of health professionals was brought home to me one day when Const and I were leaving the hospital after a therapy session. Standing in the hall between two therapy rooms, I looked up to see a big guy in hospital garb racing down the hall towards us. It took a moment for me to realize he was on an emergency call—one of the patients was in trouble. Turning the corner right behind him were more people, some in hospital uniform and some in regular dress. All of them were carrying the equipment of their special calling to provide emergency care, and they were all speeding towards their destination with determined looks on their faces.

While it was frightening to know that a life was at stake, it was comforting to be reminded of the dedication and strict adherence to procedure these people apply to helping their fellow man.

***

I am especially thankful for our health insurance, despite the costs. I was stunned when the insurance company sent me a copy of the bill they'd paid for a nine day hospital stay. It totalled nineteen thousand dollars, and from previous experience, I'm guessing it didn't include the bills for the doctors' services. And this was when Const was in for her aneurysm; I did not see the bills resulting from the care for her stroke, which included a full month's hospital stay plus four months of therapy. The costs were outrageous, but what price can you put on health?

If I have learned nothing else about caregiving, planning and maintaining a solid health insurance plan should be at the top of everyone's list. The first task is to find an insurance agent who is as interested in your problem as he is in your wallet.

If the agent says something that sounds too good to be true, it probably is. Make him put any rash statements in writing, in plain English. If he tries to change the subject when you make this request, get rid of him fast—he's not about to back up his claims. In my experience I've found that for every good agent out there, there's another one who's just one step ahead of the sheriff.

After you find an agent and insurance plan you're

satisfied with, if you find the agency doesn't aid you exactly as you expect it should, dump them as soon as you can and try another. Insurance companies can lose sight of the importance of customer service in their hurry to make money. You have to do all you can to make certain you're getting all the bang you can for your buck.

With the burgeoning costs of health services, there is definitely money to be made, and I believe that the large insurance interests have too much say in how our health care system is run. We must guard against having insurance companies decide which of the patient's needs are met and which are deemed unimportant, and try to counteract the influence they wield over our government.

For instance, the reason Const was shipped to a nursing home after being hospitalized for her broken hip was that I could not afford to pay for home care and our insurance didn't cover it. (This was unavoidable, since any plan that did include it required premiums which were too expensive for us.) A possible solution occurred to me, but I'm afraid that the way the system is set up would keep it from ever being implemented.

Why not make space available in the hospital for patients who need a minimum of nursing care? Very few hospitals have one hundred percent of their rooms filled at any one time. Rooms could be offered at a reduced rate provided the patient needed only minimum care procedures. The patient and family would be informed there would be no doctor visits except in the case of emergency, and nursing care would be restricted to perhaps two or three times a day. This service would be limited to patients who would otherwise be forced to recover under the generally inferior standards of a nursing home, and only those whom the doctor decides can fend for themselves somewhat.

Another problem that needs to be addressed is the amount of time health professionals must spend filling out forms and shuffling paperwork for the sake of insurers. In particular, I find it hard to understand why nurses are so often required to perform these chores when they should be out on the floor doing what they were trained to do. The red tape needs to be eliminated, or, if that's not possible, delegated to someone other than the person who works with the patients directly.

Every so often, usually around election time, I hear a politician bemoan the deficiencies in the U.S. health care system, but I only see them getting worse. Perhaps if our congressmen were in the same boat as other Americans, they might attack the problems more aggressively, but these legislators enjoy privileges the rest of us don't. An ambulance is always kept standing by on Capitol Hill expressly for their use, and free medical services are also available to them (the tab is picked up by you and me, of course). They're living in a glass bubble when it comes to health care, and I think it's time we broke their bubble.

With all I've said about the excellent care Const received while recovering from her health problems and how well our own insurance has served us, you may ask what I've got to complain about. I do feel fortunate for the superior level of care which my wife was given, but I have seen the problems that have plagued friends and Const's fellow patients, and have witnessed the burgeoning costs and reductions in services.

So who is ultimately to blame for the injustices of our health care system?

I am.

Voting is obviously not enough to see that needed changes are made, even when the voter makes it a point to find out from which organizations each candidate has accepted contributions. I have to monitor and talk back to elected representatives on a continual basis to let them know someone is watching them, and encourage others to do the same. Private interests like insurance companies have deep pockets and can lobby to influence government in its favor, and the only way they will be counteracted is by a big enough portion of concerned Americans making their voices heard.

Blood clots cause 75% of all strokes resulting in brain damage in the U.S., claiming 500,000 victims a year. Out of these, 150,000 are terminal cases. (These numbers are from the book *How to Prevent a Stroke*, by Peggy Jo Donahue and the editors of *Prevention* magazine, published by Rodale Press.) The mortality rate is right behind heart disease and cancer, but there is hope of improving on those numbers.

The most promising news I've heard for stroke victims comes from Malaysia. The bite of the Malaysian Pit Viper thins the blood of its victim, and at its full strength, causes internal bleeding. In smaller doses, however, it can dissolve a blood clot. Right now, its use is being concentrated on heart attack victims, but there is certainly potential for its application to strokes caused by the blockage of a blood vessel in or leading to the brain.

Considering the size of this tragedy, I can't help but feel that the Food and Drug Administration is not moving quickly enough to investigate this possible treatment, so that if it proves effective it will be available within a reasonable amount of time. While this and other drugs which have shown potential are directed through the maze of bureaucracy, you or I could be one of the next statistics.

It is my understanding that F.D.A. officials feel their organization is understaffed and underfunded, and that this may contribute to the delay in approving new treatments. When I see members of congress voting to raise their own salaries in the dark of night while the F.D.A. throws out statistics to support their argument, I can't help but think that the government's priorities have gotten out of order. While political footballs are being juggled, people like Const are suffering.

Since you're reading this book, you may have the same stake in this as I do. I hope you'll join me in letting our legislators know what's on our minds.

Fourteen
Life's Little Pleasures

There are things in life a man doesn't often discuss, but I feel it is my responsibility to help my fellow males through the difficult period caused by temporary infirmities of their spouses by exploring one of these subjects.

While a man can always go out and satisfy his appetite by purchasing this basic necessity of life, it is much more satisfying to procure it at home. While it can be a pleasure going out to a fancy place now and then, this loses its appeal after awhile.

With a little coaching, a man can continue to enjoy life's little pleasures right in the sanctity of his own residence. In fact, I've found that there are many ways to make good meals and save a lot of time in the kitchen. (You did know I was talking about cooking your own meals, didn't you?)

In the following pages I've listed some of my

favorite recipes, all of which serve two purposes. First of all, they are excellent as leftovers. If you spend too much time cooking it will soon become a mundane chore, so it is important to be able to fix something palatable which will last a couple of days. The second feature these recipes have in common is that they are all fairly easy meals to prepare. If you have looked in any cookbook you'll find that much of the stuff in there is difficult to make and some of the frills serve little use other than to decorate the table. Many of the dishes listed are often strange to the average male, and sometimes you won't find the ingredients in your local supermarket, much less in your cupboard.

I admit it: I'm a meat and potatoes man.

POTATO SOUP

Why it's called potato soup I'll never know—there are other equally important ingredients in it. Most soups can be frozen, but the potatoes have a habit of turning mushy when thawed.

Ingredients:
>   Two Potatoes
>   One Onion
>   One Can of Peas (The size depends on how well you like peas. A sixteen ounce can will do.)
>   One Pat of Butter
>   Whole Milk, or whatever is in the fridge*
>   (You'll need just enough to cover the potatoes, onion and peas.)

*It's also okay to use condensed milk diluted with water.

Peel a couple of spuds and dice them to bite size. Drop them into a pot of water as soon as possible; they turn color in short order if you don't.

Peel the onion, holding it as far enough away from you as you can to avoid having it spray into your eyes. Slice it against the grain and then cut the slices in half. (Don't chop it too small, since it'll break up more during cooking.) The size of the onion depends on how well you like them—I always use the largest one I can find.

Boil the onion and potatoes together and test the latter every now and then by fishing out a chunk and mashing it against the side of the pot using a fork. Take care not to get your sleeve too close to the fire. If the spud crushes easily, it is probably done (the potato, not your sleeve).

Open the can of peas, pour them into the colander and rinse them. (The colander is the pot with a whole lot of holes in it.) Dump the hot stuff into the colander on top of the peas and rinse.

Pour the contents of the colander back into the now-empty pot and avoid dumping any more than necessary onto the counter surface and the floor. Pour the milk over the contents (it should cover them), and set on medium heat. Add salt and pepper to taste.

Unprepared!

Drop the pat of butter into the milk and watch it closely. Once the butter has melted, the soup is ready to serve. Milk tends to foam up and make a real mess of things when heated too long, so by watching the butter in the pot you'll know when it's done without letting the milk froth.

Soda crackers or bread and butter go well with this soup. This recipe will serve one hungry man; for two people, double all the ingredients except the onion.

QUICK SPAGHETTI

Women can spend all day whipping up a batch of sauce, then spend half the night telling you why it didn't turn out. Not to fear, here's a goof-proof alternative that's easy to make.

Ingredients:
>One Pound Hamburger
>1/2 Pound Spaghetti
>1 Onion
>1/2 Green Pepper
>Mushrooms (optional) (The sliced and canned variety is fine.)
>1 Can Sliced or Whole Tomatoes, approximately 28 ounces (If whole, slice into quarters)
>1 Jar of Spaghetti Sauce, approximately 16 ounces
>1 Tablespoon Granulated Sugar (takes the sting out of tomatoes)
>Salt to taste

Slice the onion, then cut slices in half. Dice the green pepper. Fry them together with the hamburger, which you should break into small chunks, until the meat is completely browned with no pink spots showing. (If you have excess grease in the pan, drain it before going on to the next step.) Dump in the jar of spaghetti sauce and allow the mixture to simmer slowly. If you like mushrooms, now is the time to add them. Drain the juice from the tomatoes and add them to our culinary delight, then add the sugar.

Set a pot of water to boiling. Drop a pat of butter, margarine, or a teaspoon of cooking oil into the water (this will keep the spaghetti from sticking together). Add a dash of salt. (Your guess is as good as mine as to how much is in a "dash," but remember you can always add more salt later.) When the water comes to a boil, add the spaghetti and cook for about twenty minutes. Fish out a strand and squeeze it against the side of the pot, or chew it to see it it's ready. If it's tough, it needs more time.

Dig out the colander and spill the spaghetti into it and not the sink. An oven mitt or a heavy towel on the pot handle will help. Keep your face away from the contents when pouring, otherwise you'll get a blast of steam in your face.

Rinse the spaghetti in hot water. Either pour the sauce over the spaghetti or add to each plate as served. Be prepared to accept compliments from those fortunate enough to sample this cuisine. Refrigerate the leftovers, if there are any—this recipe serves two people.

HAMBURGER HOTDISH

Let me advise you up front that I hate all hotdishes except for this one.

Ingredients:
>One Pound of Hamburger
>Half a Green Pepper, diced
>One Onion, sliced and cut in half
>One Can Tomatoes (Big or small can, depending on how much you like tomatoes.)
>One Tablespoon Sugar
>Three or Four Potatoes (Again, depending on taste.)

Break up the meat into small chunks in a frying pan. Add green pepper and onion, and cook until the meat is browned. Slice potatoes and scatter the slices in the pan. (If you can, use an electric fry pan or a slow cooker, since they need less tending.) Fold in drained whole tomatoes.* Sugar removes the acid in the tomates, so add it now if you like. Season with salt and pepper to taste. Cover and cook at 350 degrees Fahrenheit for a couple hours, two should do it. To be sure it's done, stab the potatoes with a fork. If it penetrates easily, the dish is ready. This recipe will serve three people.

*"Fold in" is an expression defined in the dictionary as "to blend in a mixture, using gently cutting

strokes." In the interest of brevity, I ask you to fold in the ingredients. The sooner you do, the sooner we can eat.

DENVER SANDWICH

Don't ask me why it's called that. I think it was my dad who insisted on calling it a Denver Sandwich, and he always knew what he was talking about.

Ingredients:
> One Small Onion
> Diced Ham
> Two Eggs
> One Quarter Green Onion
> Salt and Pepper to taste
> One Teaspoon Cooking Oil

Dice onion and green pepper while warming a frying pan with a teaspoon of oil or shortening in it. Put the onion and green pepper in the pan. Load in the ham and warm it up before folding in the eggs. Stir until eggs are done. You can add salt and pepper during cooking, or after the dish is completed.

What a heck of a quick meal! Put bread and butter on the side or simply pile onto a slice of bread or toast. This is a one-serving recipe.

You may think that the above dish is just a glorified version of scrambled eggs. If so, you have a point. To make scrambled eggs, you'd leave out the ham, green pepper and onion, and add about a teaspoonful of milk to the above.

VEGETABLE BEEF SOUP

This is another of my favorites and very easy to fix. It's good left over, but I suggest you remove the potatoes if you want to freeze it.

A handy way to get most of the ingredients for this dish already chopped up and mixed together is to buy packages of "stew vegetables" or "mixed vegetables" in the frozen food section of your grocery store. Throw them in right out of the package—they'll thaw as the soup simmers. Most people have a special fondness for fresh vegetables, though, so I've used them in this recipe.

Ingredients:
> One Pound Stew Meat, rinsed and diced
> Two or Three Potatoes, depending on personal preference
> One Large Onion
> Three of Four Carrots
> One Can of Peas (optional)
> 1/2 Teaspoon Salt
> 1/4 Teaspoon Pepper

When dicing up the stew meat, it is helpful to have it partially frozen; it cuts more easily that way. Dice into about 1/4 inch cubes for best results. Dump into a dry pot (the pot should have a capacity of at least a half gallon) under full heat and stir frequently with a wooden spoon. Do not be disturbed at the resulting coating on the sides and bottom of the pot. When cooking, this will serve to flavor and color the soup. Fry until the meat is fully browned.

Add water to the pot, enough to cover the ingredients while keeping the liquid a lusty brown. It will fizzle for a moment before settling down. Remember, the more water you use, the more salt you'll need to add. Taste test to keep control; I usually add more water by the glass when required. This is a good time to put in the salt and pepper. I've been pretty conservative with it because the soup can always be seasoned to taste by the individual, so don't be insulted if they reach for the salt shaker.

Cut the onions into rather large chunks for the convenience of the guests who don't like onions. (They will probably hide them under the soup dish.) Peel and dice potatoes into large chunks for the same reason.

If you like peas, open the can, drain and rinse before throwing them into the pot. For that matter, the adventurous chefs out there can toss in anything else laying around that looks like it belongs. (They might want to check with the other people who will be eating the soup before getting too creative, however.)

Once it begins to boil, turn down the heat and simmer for an hour or so until the spuds can be speared easily with a fork.

The soup is best if allowed to cool down and reheated. This recipe will serve three to four people, and leftovers can be frozen. (You might want to eat all of the potatoes first, though, as the spuds get mushy when thawed.)

VEGETABLE STEW

This is just like the vegetable soup, except the peas are mandatory and the stew needs to be thickened.

Thickening: You can use either flour or cornstarch to thicken stew gravy. I prefer cornstarch, since it's easier to work with. Mix up about a half cup of cold water with two teaspoons of cornstarch in a separate container, preferably a glass jar with a cover or a measuring cup. Add salt and pepper—three shakes of pepper and six or eight of salt should do it. Stir it some more. It is more important to get the lumps out than to worry about the consistency; thickening will take care of itself when the liquid is added to the kettle of delectables, which should be done when the vegetables are soft. Pour slowly into the pot and stir with the big wooden spoon you used to threaten the kids with. The stuff will thicken slowly, but remember to turn off the heat before it gets to the proper viscosity— it will continue to thicken by itself.

ROASTS

Now that you've gotten some experience under your belt and are probably hungry for something more substantial, let's try a roast. Maybe even go for a real delight, beef and pork roasts cooked together. If you are a gravy lover, you'll love the combination.

The size of the meat depends on the number of guests or how well you like cold leftovers. In any case, I suggest you use about half the amount of pork as beef. Plan for about a half pound of meat per person. Wash off the meat to remove bone chips and the butcher's fingerprints. I prefer to use an electric skillet to cook in, since I find the meat tastes better, but you can use a gas or electric oven too.

Always put the pork roast in first—it takes longer to cook and pork should always be well done. First, brown all sides of the meat in a frying pan to make it more appealing and to help flavor the gravy. Place the roast in an oven pan at 375 degrees, season with salt and pepper, then lay thick slices of onion on top. (If you're using an electric skillet you can use it for both browning and roasting, leaving one less pan to wash —another reason I like using one.)

After about a half hour, give the beef roast the same treatment, put it in the same oven pan as the pork and add about a cup of water before going to read the funnies. Be sure to pour the water around the meat instead of over it, so you don't wash the seasonings off. Turn both roasts over after about a half hour, and add more water if the pan is dry. The important thing to watch is the amount of water in the pan; you'll probably scorch the meat and smell up the kitchen if it's neglected. Even if that happens, however, don't worry—just turn the meat over and re-water it. Once the pork comes apart easily with a fork, you know it's done, and so is the beef.

Make gravy with the drippings on the stovetop, after removing the meat from the pan. Mix about a tablespoon of cornstarch and a half cup of cold water in a separate container. Stir thoroughly to avoid lumps, and shake in some salt and pepper. Turn the heat up under the pan and work the shreds of browned meat from the bottom and edges with a tablespoon, then slowly pour in your cornstarch and water mixture, stirring the whole time. When your gravy gets a little thinner than you'd prefer, then turn off the heat. Remember, it'll get thicker by itself.

You might as well enjoy some baked potatoes with your meal. Just wash them, stick them with a fork (to keep them from blowing up) and put them in the oven when you put in the roast. Wrapping them in aluminum foil is optional—I find I like them better without it. (If you're using an electric cooker, they can go right in the pan.) I realize you could microwave the potatoes for five to ten minutes instead, but if you love the skins, baking is better.

RIBS AND KRAUT

You don't have to be German to enjoy them, but it probably helps.

Ingredients:
>One Pound Spare Ribs
>One Can Sauerkraut, approximately 28 ounces
>One Teaspoon Caraway Seed
>Two Tablespoons Brown Sugar

Wash ribs and put in a slow cooker with very little water, about two tablespoons. Heap on the sauerkraut and sprinkle the seeds and brown sugar over the top. Let them steep all day if you find it convenient, but they should cook until the meat is falling off the bones. (The brown sugar takes a lot of the zing out of the kraut; if you like the zing, leave it out.) Serves three people.

AMERICAN POTATO SALAD

In so far as I am concerned, it is very easy to avoid screwing up potato salad. But boy, can some people screw it up!

Ingredients:
>Six Medium-sized Potatoes
>One Onion
>One Half Green Pepper

Unprepared!

One Teaspoon Pimento (optional; it's mostly for color, not taste)
One Tablespoon Milk
A Few Drops (about a quarter teaspoon) Cider Vinegar, White Vinegar, or Lemon Juice
Salt and Pepper to Taste
One Teaspoon Sugar, if desired
One Cup Salad Dressing (I prefer it to mayonnaise)

Use new potatoes if possible (the ones with red skins). The others are alright, too, but aren't as flavorful. Boil potatoes until done, using the crushing or spearing tests.

Allow potatoes to cool until firm before trying to peel them. It helps to wash the residue off the peeler or paring knife periodically. (The special flavoring in the salad comes from boiling them with the skins on.) Dice them, along with the onion, green pepper, and pimento. Fold in pimento, green pepper and onion with diced potatoes and let stand while mixing the dressing.

Put the salad dressing in a small bowl. Add approximately one tablespoon of milk, a few shakes of salt and pepper, no more than six drops of vinegar (cider or white, or better yet, some lemon juice). Mix until smooth. Taste test the mixture before adding to the potatoes. Probably needs a little more salt or some sugar if it tastes sharp or too tangy.

Pour some onto the potatoes and mix in. When all the spuds have a thin coating, you might want to add a sliced boiled egg and/or a sliced red radish as a garnish. But if you're very hungry, don't worry about how it looks.

TUNA FISH SALAD

Ingredients:

> One Six Ounce Can of Tuna, Packed in Water
> 1/2 Pound of Macaroni Shells
> 1/2 Medium Size Onion
> 1/4 Green Pepper
> One Can of Peas, approximately 16 ounces
> One Cup Dressing (see American Potato Salad recipe)
> Pepper, Celery Salt, Onion Powder, and Garlic Powder (as seasonings)
> Salt to taste

In a pot of water, bring shells to a boil using our old trick of adding a little butter or cooking oil to keep them from sticking together. Toss in about six shakes of salt to season once they have come to a boil. When done, empty the macaroni into our old friend the colander and rinse well.

Dice up the onion and green pepper and fold into the shells. (See what a useful word "fold" is?) Put the mixture into a large serving bowl, unless you have a spare colander, since we need one for the rest of the job. Open the can of tuna and put it in the colander; break up the chunks into smaller pieces. Be sure to give it a good healthy rinse. Once drained, put the tuna into the salad bowl with the other ingredients.

Put peas into the colander, and, you got it, rinse them, drain, and fold into shell mix. Then use the salad dressing recipe from our American Potato Salad and mix it in; about a cup will do, but don't overwhelm the concoction.

Now is the time for the seasonings, and much of this is a matter of personal taste. For instance, if garlic powder warps your taste buds, use very little or none at all. Keep tasting as you go along, but remember that celery salt is the key to bringing out the flavor. Don't be shaken by its color; it is an off brown, not white or green as you might expect. The seasoning salts do not have to be mixed separately—just sprinkle each one on the top of the salad and mix everything together. Or, you can put them out on the table and leave it up to your guests to season their own portions themselves. This recipe serves four.

One last tip: this salad improves if left refrigerated overnight. You may have to add more dressing when you serve it, however, as it tends to dry out a bit.

A FEW PARTING TIPS

Fried Potatoes: If you're tired of peeling potatoes before frying them, wash them thoroughly and slice them with the skins on. They can be enhanced by adding diced onions or green peppers, either before or after the spuds are cooked.

Pancakes: Go ahead and follow the recipe on the box, but dig out the cornflakes and throw a handful into the batter. This really adds to the flavor, tastes kind of nutty. You can experiment with the amount according to your taste.

Bratwurst: You can grill or fry brats. They are done just before they start to burst out of their skins. Keep rotating them on the grill until you give them a nice tan. In the fry pan, you can cover them with water or beer and allow them to simmer, and when the water/beer is used up, you begin to turn them until a tasty looking color appears. You can also soak the brats in beer overnight for an extra special flavor, then cook them in the same beer. I wouldn't try to drink the leftover liquid, though.

Okay, so maybe you won't qualify as a chef at the Waldorf once you've mastered these simple recipes, but you'll be able to keep some meat on your bones. I haven't divulged some of my best kept secrets for a very simple reason: Your wife is going to wonder where you got all the cooking knowledge as it is—I wouldn't want to be responsible for you winding up as your household's only cook for the rest of your life. All I wanted to do was make sure you don't starve.

Fifteen

Looking Towards the Future

In looking after the queen, I neglected a primary rule for caregivers: don't ignore your own health while you focus your attention on someone else's.

My shoulder had been bothering me for about five months before I did anything about it. I knew I had strained it by constantly helping Const out of the wheelchair, bed, davenport and the like, and was waiting for the pain and discomfort to go away by itself. The only problem was that it hadn't improved in all that time. What I didn't know was that my shoulder strain had turned into bursitis.

Bursitis can perhaps best be described as a freezing up of the joint. The ache it produces is unbelievable, but fortunately it can be cleared up in a variety of ways. Special exercises may be called for, or a cortisone shot might help. Having the joint manipulated while the patient is under anaesthesia is yet another method of dealing with the problem.

In my case, my doctor prescribed exercises, and they seemed to help, but I discovered a round of golf helped a lot more. The lesson I learned from the experience is that if you don't take care of yourself, you can easily go from being a caregiver to being on the receiving end of the care.

I now pay more attention to my own health, and I try to always keep a positive attitude. Fortunately, we do not know how things will end in the short term. Const remains fearful of another stroke, and has repeatedly told me she does not know if she would be able to handle it. Her medication and the watchful eye of her doctor are the only safeguards against it happening again.

I refuse to dwell on this. For all I know, I could be next, and you can't live your life worrying about what might happen. I just hope that they don't have washing machines and vacuum cleaners in the next world.

Our lives are taken up with more immediate concerns, and I've found that in order to manage all the things that must be done, a written schedule is very helpful. I like to put a sheet of paper on the cupboard and jot down things to be done for the day, the week, or whenever I get around to it. I've heard it called a "honey do" sheet, as in "honey do this, honey do that." The size of the list can be discouraging at first, but suddenly you find most of the things are crossed off. Don't worry about getting bored, though—you can always add new projects. Being a maverick, I changed the name of the list from a "honey do" list to a "melon" list. (You know, like in "Honey Dew Melons.")

My cat Sam began to do his part to make sure I got an early start on things. He took to stepping on the alarm on our clock radio every morning at about three o'clock. While I am in the habit of rising early, I didn't need him to hustle me out of bed any earlier. Const was not at all pleased with his new trick, either. Since I was the one who brought Sam home, she does not bother to distinguish between his bad habits and mine.

But her reaction was good; it was yet another indication of her getting better. When she was almost helpless, I pretty much ran things my own way, but as she improved, things started to change.

This is a phase in the recovery of a stroke victim I touched upon when describing Const's initial recovery period, but which I feel needs to be covered in greater depth.

For over a year, I had taken on the responsibility for all household chores. Some of them I didn't mind, and others were distasteful to me. No matter what I thought of these tasks, however, I did them because they needed to be done.

As Const grew stronger and more assertive, she began to supervise me more closely. I had to swallow a lot of pride and bite my tongue while being trained to do things her way, even though she was generally right. Functioning at about seventy percent of her old health, she was maneuvering around using the vacuum as a cane and countertops in lieu of her walker. She was surpassing the progress made before her fall, becoming independent once again.

Upon her becoming more active, however, I found it just didn't work for both of us to try to cooperate on any single chore other than making the bed. One or the other of us would do the dishes; I was far too impatient to stand by while she washed, waiting to dry them. For her part, she seemed happy to have an increasing share of the household work back as her sole domain.

I could see the handwriting on the wall: the chief cook and bottle washer was well on the way to losing his job. This did not bother me in the least.

During the time I'd taken care of the housekeeping by myself, I learned a great deal about things I'd never had any inclination to study, but which I can now fully appreciate. I had always known Const had invested a lot of time and effort on my behalf, and had looked upon her stroke as my turn to pay those dues, in a manner of speaking. But you know what? I'm proud of having handled those responsibilities. I derived real satisfaction from keeping the household running, from the accomplishment of something as small as putting together an edible meal. And while she was regaining her role as homemaker, I had become cognizant of the extent of her duties and more aware of when I should pitch in.

From being a totally helpless individual with complete loss of arm, hand, leg and foot movement, she could now stand and walk, climb stairs, wash dishes, peel potatoes, and perform many other tasks. Of course, there were still things too difficult to manage. Putting up her hair, cutting meat, and some other chores requiring both hands were yet to be conquered. But when she couldn't coax her left hand to help, she constantly tried ways to do things one handed. This determination to do for herself has been a great factor in her recovery.

As far as her hip injury is concerned, recent x-rays showed that in spite of some continuing discomfort, all was in place and generally copacetic. Her doctor assured her that everything was fine, and told her in a nice way that she had very little padding on her hips to reduce the discomfort she was feeling. I hoped that this would help convince her she didn't need to be concerned about her weight, but we shall see. In any case, the big challenge remains her rehabilitation from the stroke.

Connie Shaffer's description of how the brain can find alternate routes when the old ones are blocked certainly rang true based on my observations. The comparison which makes most sense to me is that the brain is like a warship: if the steering is shot out on one side of the ship, another set of steering apparatus is usable on the other side. The brain only needs to be shown there is another way of doing things.

As Const progressed, I was reminded of a child learning to do something. A stroke victim not only needs to know what must be done, but his or her brain needs to be taught and the muscles must be conditioned through constant work and practice.

Our church installed an elevator to help handicapped people. It only goes up one flight, so I have to admire them for putting it in. I encourage Const not to use it, which is fine by her; the steps are among the

189

best forms of therapy for her. Our own basement steps are relatively short and are carpeted, so they do not lend themselves to stair climbing practice. The church steps are deeper, polished, and have a sturdy handrail. She almost licks her chops at the challenge.

Almost invariably, when we start going up them, someone rushes up and informs us about the elevator. Const knows they are well intentioned, so she smiles and takes the time to tell them she is aware of it, but wants the therapy.

One of the most difficult things for Const to admit, however, was that she could no longer crochet or knit. She used to teach these skills, and one day she will again, this I know. In the meantime, this isn't something I can help her with. (To me, crochet hooks are only good for picking the meat out of nuts.) She instead contented herself with making stitched designs on scarves and tablecloths; this activity is not her first love, but it satisfied some of the creative urges in her. And while it was difficult for me to watch her frustrated attempts at needlework, the important thing was that she tried. There is no pot of gold at the top of the mountain, and you and I know the real challenge is in the climb.

---

*In the National Stroke Association's book, **The Road Ahead: A Stroke Recovery Guide**, it is pointed out that dwelling on what life could have been like if the stroke hadn't happened only feeds into the depression process. The healthy alternative is for the caregiver and stroke survivor to create new goals for their lives. The goals may be in such areas as physical rehabilita-*

tion, social and recreational needs, and their family and community. It is helpful to establish both short and long term goals, and plan activities that will serve as steps in accomplishing the goals.

The changes that stroke brings can create many challenges. Working through the challenges in a positive, constructive, and systematic manner helps to ease tension and bring about solutions more readily. When the person is confronted with a problem, it is necessary to first acknowledge and identify it as being problematic. It is then useful to identify why this is a problem, and what causes could have contributed to it. The next task is to determine what the desired end result is and to come up with possible ways to achieve it. After reviewing the options for solutions, the person chooses the one that best meets his or her needs and identifies the behaviors that will carry out the chosen solution. In understanding and practicing basic problem solving techniques, the individual will feel more confident and successful in conquering the challenges that the stroke has brought on.

The impact of stroke is multidimensional, affecting areas of the individual's physical, psychological, and social life. By developing a better understanding of stroke and the impact that it can have, the stroke survivor and the caregiver can become better equipped to meet the challenges, and work together to create a more positive and productive recovery process.

At the time of this writing, Const is doing well, impatient as ever to get over this thing. We have learned to settle for small accomplishments, and I keep reminding her a lot of little things add up to big things. Our experience shows her this is true.

A couple of nights ago, sitting on the divan, she tried to reach up and put her hand behind her head. The first try got the hand about shoulder high, and nowhere near the target. The second try was a slight improvement.

"That trip was better," I pressed.

"I'll never get better."

"Try it once more," I said.

She struggled valiantly, and slowly her hand traveled up to shoulder level, then behind her neck. Suddenly a smile spread over her face as she shrieked, "I'm touching the other ear!"

That was quite a milestone for us, but an even more momentous one was passed yesterday. You might remember my explaining how I felt that her fall was due to her inability to walk with a normal heel-toe effort.

Out of the blue, with the aid of her walker, she was able to place her heel down first! After seventeen months of trying, she finally did it.

Way to go, baby. We're winning this war.

The Contributors

Mary Hughes, M.A. is a licensed Social Worker who holds a Masters Degree in Counseling Psychology and a Bachelors Degree in Social Work. She has had twelve years of experience working in the human service field, with an emphasis on helping older adults and persons suffering from acute or chronic illnesses. For the past five years, Mary has worked at Fairview Southdale Hospital in Edina, Minnesota as a Medical Social Worker on the neurological, gerontological, medical and pediatric units. She also works with Fairview Southdale's Outpatient Mental Health Program, providing individual and group therapy. Throughout Mrs. Collins' recovery, she and her husband Ellwyn have been active members of Fairview Southdale's Stroke Support Group, which Mary co-facilitates.

Constance Saathoff Shaffer, O.T.R. graduated from Mount Mary College in Milwaukee, Wisconsin in 1985 with a B.S. in Occupational Therapy. After finishing school she took a position at Baptist Hospital in Nashville, Tennessee, where she worked in Acute Care and in the Rehabilitation Center with patients suffering from spinal cord injuries, cardiovascular accidents, arthritis, joint replacements, and head injuries. She moved to Minneapolis, Minnesota in 1989 and began working at Fairview Southdale Hospital. In 1991 she left the hospital setting, and is now employed in an Industrial Rehabilitation Clinic at Park Nicollet Medical Center, where she works with people who have been injured on the job and are in need of reconditioning in order to return to their places of employment.

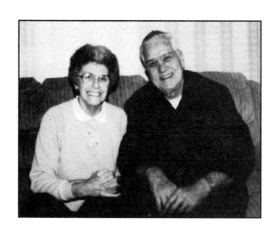

About the Author

Ellwyn K. Collins, pictured above with his wife
Constance, lives in Bloomington, Minnesota, where
Mrs. Collins continues to progress in her recovery
from stroke. When she first fell ill, Mr. Collins looked
for a book which would offer support in dealing with
the multitude of changes occurring in his life. Unable
to find one written from a male perspective, he
decided to write *Unprepared!* This is Mr. Collins' first
book.

About the Author